The
Fearless
Pregnancy

Transition from Your Fertility
Journey to "Mama to Be" with Ease,
Joy, and Unshakable Confidence

ROSANNE AUSTIN

Published 2022

ISBN 979-8-9873031-1-5 (paperback)

ISBN 979-8-9873031-0-8 (eBook)

Proofread: Megan Harris, www.mharriseditor.com

Author Photo: Wendy K. Yalom

CONTENTS

- when you feel afraid, talk to this baby
  "mum gets a bit scog, anxious but you
  are safe, can't wait to meet you"
- Don't worry
- You are coming to this family and we
  are all excited
- Can't wait to get to know you
- can't wait to show you....xxx
- can't wait for you to wear the hiking bag

Want a FREE cheat sheet with my Fearless Pregnancy Fear-Neutralizing Tools?

Let's put my very best tools at your fingertips so you can live your miracle pregnancy with ease, joy, and unshakable confidence!

As a big thank you for including this book in your pregnancy journey, I want to give you a quick and easy way to refer to the tools I share in this book for the moments when you *really* need them.

No need to try to remember *where* they are in the book— I've got you, boo.

This is the perfect complement to your healthy, happy pregnancy.

Save your cheat sheet to your phone or print it and tuck it into your bag.

Either way, these tools will be there for you!

Get your *free* Fearless Pregnancy Cheat Sheet NOW!

Scan the QR code or go to https://www.frommaybetobaby.com/ffp-gift-1.

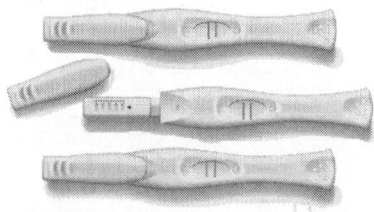

Chapter 1

You Made It to the "Other Side." Welcome!

Mama, the fact that you are reading this makes me guess that something truly magical has happened in your life: *you are pregnant!*

To the rest of the world, getting pregnant might not seem like a big enough deal to call it "magical"—it happens for women every day and is seen as "a given"—but this book is not written for the "rest of the world." Unlike whatever "they" might expect, when *you* saw those two pink lines on a pregnancy test or the word "pregnant" in bold, it felt neither "everyday" nor like "a given." For you, getting to this baby was a journey, filled with tears, uncertainty, incredible highs, heartbreaking lows, moments of desperation, bouts of despair, and mind-bending existential questions. You and I get to squeal with excitement that you made it *here*.

(Take a moment to let a glee-filled girly *"Eeeek!"* escape your lips if that feels awesome.)

Chances are, you picked up this book after a long fertility journey, one that you hope has finally come to the happily-ever-after ending you've longed for. (I know the word "long" is relative, but let's be honest: any amount of time you spent in fear that this baby wouldn't show up can feel like forever!)

Together we are going to zero in on a very specific issue, one that is rarely acknowledged, much less discussed: *Now that I've finally gotten my big fat positive (aka BFP), how do I not drive myself crazy and worry myself sick for the next forty weeks? I'm so happy I'm pregnant, but at the same time, I'm scared something could happen and take all of this away.*

To the outside world, once you get your BFP, your world "should" be turned into a series of joyful mama-to-be diaper commercials with nothing but daisies, butterflies, and gauzy scenes from boho pregnancy shoots. Not so much for women like us who struggled with fertility. Our stories of making our way to the baby aisles at our local big box stores were more nail-biters than they were breezy beach reads, so skipping over *that* reality and diving straight into the mechanics of "what comes next" feels woefully lacking. After months and years of living in fear that "it" might not ever happen, it's like whiplash to make a hard right turn out of survival mode into the peachy-keen, happily-ever-after daydream people might expect. We are bruised and battle-weary, and we just want to know it's finally safe to put down the sword. *(Just writing those words takes me back!)* Don't worry, Mama, by the end of this book, you'll understand that it's safe to put that weapon away and let your fighting days be a thing of the past.

PICKING UP THIS BOOK WAS REALLY SMART

Instead of glossing over your fertility journey like it didn't happen, like it was a mere blip on your radar screen and your BFP has taken all your cares away, we are going to do something way smarter. Throughout this book, I am going to share tools, strategies, and ideas that are going to help you thoughtfully navigate this exciting (and sometimes scary) time in your life. Acknowledging your worries about how this precious pregnancy is going to play out is way more productive than pretending they aren't there or trying to hide them under a brittle veneer of being all smiles, then going right back to being terrified of seeing blood the next time you pee. *(If that little bit of truth caught your attention, then buckle up, sister. There's more where that came from —and I have a really cool tool to help you with that exact issue!)*

What I will be sharing will apply to your pregnancy, regardless of whether it's your first baby or you are completing your family. My goal is to empower women during their pregnancy miracles, regardless of how many times they've been on this merry-go-round and no matter how high the odds are stacked against them.

Let me first acknowledge that if you are both excited and scared, that is perfectly okay. Having lived a fertility journey means that you have a unique appreciation for what's at stake. Maybe this baby is the result of repeated fertility treatments after many invasive interventions—or maybe they were a natural miracle after all seemed lost. Whatever the case may be, this pregnancy is special. You and your partner aren't that couple who just looked at each other and got pregnant. You had to go to lengths that others didn't. You may have even taken your relationship and lifestyle to their limits to get here. Well done! And your situation is unique; therefore, the way you feel today requires a specialized approach and journey-tested, miracle-pregnancy-oriented solutions. This is exactly why I am so

4 | ROSANNE AUSTIN

excited you have this book in your hands. In no uncertain terms, *I can help you*, just as I have helped thousands of women around the world.

YOU CAN BE 100% SURE YOU'RE IN GOOD HANDS

Here's why this book is worthy of your time and attention: after seven years of failed fertility treatments and one heartbreaking miscarriage (with the last of our embryos), my husband and I conceived our son, Asher, naturally when I was almost forty-three. Because I was in my forties with a shoddy fertility past, everyone around me, including my doctor, was on high alert. And I admit, when I saw the two pink lines on my pregnancy test, I was elated beyond belief, but my mind also immediately went into overdrive with fear for my baby: *Will he make it this time? I did this naturally… I have so little information! Can't I just skip ahead to the delivery room scene so I can finally hold him in my arms?* All of that flashed through my mind in milliseconds. But thankfully, the mindset work I had done prior to my miracle pregnancy (spoiler alert: more on this later!) empowered me to move out of fear and into Mama Bear mode (more on this later, too!).

Rest assured that I didn't just wake up one day enlightened and fully at peace on my journey. It was work. I was fighting decades of programming that told me that I was unworthy of the good I truly desired, that "having it all" was for other people, and that following my heart wasn't enough. Past Me had blown off anything having to do with "mindset" as woo-woo nonsense. I hadn't thought I needed that "stuff"… until, of course, the pain of my journey brought me to my knees. At the time, I was a career prosecutor, taking sexual assault cases to trial. I was in a profession that worships logic *("Just the facts, ma'am.")* and celebrates an almost pathological fixation with "worst-case scenarios" as proof of good case preparation. (Back in the day, I'd be able to give you a list of eye-watering worst-case scenarios that would put Chicken Little to shame and have you wondering if I was in need of professional help. But I digress.) At the time, I believed that medicine alone could save me... until it didn't.

I quickly realized that something needed to change—and that something was me. But I didn't know how or what to change, so I did two insanely smart things: I began to study, and I asked for help. I read countless books, attended dozens of seminars, invested hundreds of thousands of dollars in hiring the best mentors in the world (no joke), and consistently practiced the principles that I now teach. What I did not only changed my life, but it also, in no uncertain terms, helped bring my son to me at a time when I had no reason to believe that was possible. I promise you that I am probably one of the most stubborn women you will ever meet, and if *I* was able to change, I know you can, too.

This is why, when it comes to helping women put the mindset piece of the fertility puzzle in place so they can finally get (and stay) pregnant, I'm not guessing, nor am I just parroting something I read about in a book. I lived it myself, and *I wrote the book.* Over my past eight years of coaching women to fertility success, my clients, ranging from ages twenty-eight to fifty-two, have beaten some of the most harrowing odds. Some have even had a less than 1% chance of ever conceiving by any means, but then, once they added what I teach to the mix, *Boom! Pregnant.* With all of these successes, my clients very quickly began banging down my door to help with what they saw as the next (albeit delightful) "problem."

My clients began asking me to coach them through their pregnancies. They saw the dramatic way in which mindset had supported their success in getting pregnant and they wanted to keep the goodness of that momentum going. As soon as those two lines showed up, they understood they'd be facing an entirely new set of concerns. It's one thing to pray for a moment to come, but it's another to know exactly how to move through it with peace, confidence, and resilience when it arrives. The pressure can be intense, and past heartbreaks or disappointments can steal the well-deserved joy from the moment. Having lived both sides of this journey, I was (and am) honored to take up the challenge and show my Miracle Mamas all I had learned.

When my clients started using the set of pregnancy tools I created for them, they began moving through the most challenging times of their respective pregnancies with the expectation of success, ease, and—wait for it—joy! *This. This is why I wrote this book.* I wrote this book so that women who struggled with their fertility could make the leap from *trying* to be moms to *being moms* with the peace they have so dearly earned.

I want every Miracle Mama who refuses to settle for forty weeks of fear to have the support she needs to start each day with confidence, to know how to approach the anxiety-laden early weeks of her miracle pregnancy with ease, and to have a practical tool kit for dealing with the unique stressors that show up for women who have lived this journey.

THE FEARLESS PREGNANCY: OUR SHARED GOAL

The primary goal of this book is to help you be Fearless during this pregnancy. You've come so far that you deserve to enjoy every last moment of it without fear. In what I brand as "The Fearless Pregnancy," it's all about swapping out your fear for the blissful, Mama Bear energy that you deserve to feel, having worked so hard to get "here." The Fearless Pregnancy is not just a mindset, it's about the actions you take—and how you show up in the world—as you navigate the next forty-ish weeks.

What I will be sharing in this book is a road map and a reference for you to use during your pregnancy. Having been "there" myself and having walked countless clients through this process, I know how excited (and scared) you may be. Rest assured,

Mama, that with this book in your hands, you are definitely in the right place.

The Fearless Pregnancy is an ethos, a way of being. Its most notable characteristic is an unwavering belief that the desire in your heart to be a mom was meant for you. Therefore, this pregnancy is not "luck," and no matter what shows up, *you know* how this story ends: you will have a baby in your arms. If this sounds like one hell of a double scoop of confidence, you are absolutely right. But don't be fooled. It's not hubris. It's trust— in yourself and the Universe that brought you this baby. That is the kind of confidence that is not only real, but sustainable.

I realize that this may sound like a stretch, but I will be teaching you, step by step, what needs to be done to cultivate this belief. When you have it, you will be able to step up to any twist, turn, challenge, or surprise that shows up during your pregnancy with a level of ease and expectation that the highest good will be done. You don't have to spend the next forty-something weeks in terror, waiting for the other shoe to drop, or wondering if you will wake from this blissful dream. This dream is your new life. Making your dreams your reality is your new normal.

Embracing The Fearless Pregnancy will give you a skill set that will serve you, not just now, but well after you have this precious baby, and ultimately in every aspect of your life. I say that with Fearless Confidence because I see this truth playing out in the lives of my ladies day in and day out. Not only do they call in their miracle pregnancies, but they also go on to dramatically advance in their careers, deepen their relationships, start thriving businesses, and create lives that they thought were only for "other people." You can hear some of them tell their stories on my *Fearlessly Fertile* podcast, as well as on my YouTube channel, *Fearlessly Fertile with Rosanne Austin*. Their results speak for themselves.

The Fearless Pregnancy isn't about denying your (possibly)

well-founded fears or concerns. Fearlessness is not the absence of fear. It describes the way you approach fear when it shows up. And, unquestionably, it *will* show up. But don't worry; you will be well prepared.

OUR ROAD MAP FORWARD

Each chapter in this book will move through a chronological progression of stages in your pregnancy and specifically address the mindset shifts that will support you to live it Fearlessly. From the moment that you find out you are pregnant to your preparation for your delivery, I've gotchu, boo. You will have tools, strategies, and thorough explanations for what I am presenting you with each teaching and why. I have also included specific stories of my clients who implemented what I taught and are now holding their babies because of it.

Each chapter includes relevant exercises to help you deepen your understanding and to give you a practical application for the concepts presented. And, to make this book even more useful to you, I've given you a summary of all the tools at the end so that, when you have a "break glass in case of emergency" moment, you will know exactly where to turn. You will be surrounded with support and uplifting examples of why being Fearless during your pregnancy is one of the best decisions you will ever make. By the end of this book, you will have a full arsenal of ways to keep yourself focused, confident, and at peace during your pregnancy, which you certainly deserve.

As you read this book, give yourself plenty of grace, as perhaps some of the concepts I present may be new, while others may be more familiar. In either case, give yourself the chance to onboard these ideas from the new perspective you have as a pregnant lady.

Even if this isn't your first pregnancy, you've never been in this exact moment before, with this exact pregnancy. Refuse to let the past cast a shadow on what's possible for you now, in this time.

It is with so much excitement and love in my heart that I invite you to receive the hard-won wisdom I have to share in the pages ahead.

Congratulations, Mama. Here's to your Fearless Pregnancy.

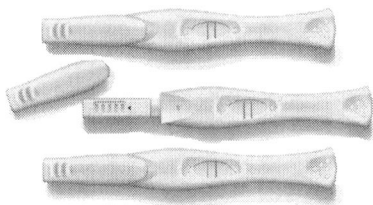

Chapter 2

Wait... I'm Pregnant?

It's a funny thing to finally get what you want. When you've been in chase-the-dream-mode for what seems like an eternity, seeing those two lines on your pregnancy test can be an odd mix of elation and confusion. Yes, you see the two lines, you understand what they mean, but at the same time, you're thinking, "Wait. *Me?*"

If you are anything like I was, in those milliseconds when your mind is racing to catch up with what your eyes perceive on the test, it's as if the world goes quiet and time slows down, and it feels like your head is about to explode. You wonder if your vision is failing you or if your "journey fatigue" has caused you to slip into a wishful-thinking fertility mirage. But, deep down, you know exactly what you are seeing. *You know*. You feel a primal scream forming from the depths of your soul, your eyes well up with tears, and your otherwise advanced vocabulary turns into a tongue-tied, garbled mess. And, when the words you prayed to utter form in your mind and cross your lips, you feel the invisible weight you've been carrying during your entire fertility journey lift, even if momentarily, from your body.

I'M PREGNANT!

Yes, Mama, yes you are. This is a moment that will be emblazoned on your heart forever—not just because it's the moment you realize you are pregnant, but because it feels like you can finally step off the "trying to conceive" crazy train. You made it!

I'M PREGNANT... GULP!

There is an interesting phenomenon that occurs, however, particularly in my never-slow-down women who've spent some time on this journey. Once the initial excitement of being able to tell your husband or partner and anyone else you want to share this glorious news with hits its peak, you find yourself at a tipping point where the glee begins to slide right into the awkward embrace of a question that not many of us are prepared to answer: *Now what?*

It doesn't matter how long you have fantasized about this moment or how intricately you daydreamed about every possible scenario. This question will show up, tapping its toe and fidgeting, as it awaits your answer—while you stand there with a lump in your throat, stumped.

Pregnancy seemed like such a far-off, incredibly exclusive destination that you weren't always 100% sure you'd ever get "there." Perhaps you figured that when you got to Baby Bump Island, it would just be a never-ending, steady stream of victory parades and confetti raining down from the heavens for forty weeks. Well, you are here now, sister, so let me give you some basics for navigating this pivotal moment in your life so you can wisely answer that sneaky Saboteur question. (Note: If you are unfamiliar with what I mean when I say "Saboteur," that is simply a term I learned from the Coaches Training Institute. It describes our negative, fearful, inner voice that inspires self-doubt, worry, and, well, a pattern of self-sabotage! We all have it, and we've all found ourselves in the clutches of our Saboteurs in one way or another. And, just so you know, there's usually more than one. Totally normal! And now you have a name for that voice that fits it to a T.)

First, I want you to understand that you don't have to rush to "know" or answer the question. The wisest thing you can do for yourself and your baby in this moment is to simply be in the excitement and joy of this time. "Now what?" may feel like a familiar mindset; it's a question that we all constantly asked ourselves during our fertility journeys to bring some semblance of order to what felt like chaos. It's a fear-based demand to know what comes next, to create the illusion of predictability and certainty on a journey that was, by its very nature, devoid of either. In this precious stage, when you find out that your baby is here, you don't have to *do* anything—you get to *be*. Excited, grateful, relieved, humbled, scared, amazed, unsure, blown away, surprised, and any other states of being that show up. You've spent years praying to get to this place, so don't worry about this question; it will be answered soon enough.

I know that even as you read this, your Saboteurs will keep hammering you with "Now what?" and will try to rush you out of this bliss, but tell them to pipe down for now. We will return to this question later in this chapter.

YES, YOU DESERVE THIS

Having lived this journey myself and having coached women around the world through their pregnancies, I know a question that runs neck and neck with "Now what?" is one that goes something like this: "Am I really worthy of receiving this good in my life?"

This is a distinctly different sensation than the initial disbelief we might have when we first see those two lines on the pregnancy test. This speaks to the core of what we believe about ourselves and whether we are deserving of finally seeing our dream unfold before our eyes. While I've devoted an entire chapter to the incredibly important topic of "receiving," suffice it to say here that it's totally okay to receive the gift of this pregnancy. You get to have this blessing in your life!

This idea may be hard for you to believe right now, and if that is the case, go ahead and borrow a cup of my faith. Having spent the last eight years of my life watching women make their mom dreams come true, I have plenty of it.

There is something the women in my Fearlessly Fertile community know me for, aside from my pink hair and enthusiastic use of expletives. It is a simple but definitive statement of faith: "The desire in your heart to be a mom is there because it was meant for you." Now that you have seen the two lines, Mama, this statement takes on a new and even more important role. Your prayers have been answered. Your intention has been made manifest. Embrace it. When a desire is truly from your heart and your intentions are clean and not motivated by fear, lack, or scarcity, a way will be found, and victory is an inevitability. You are here. Everything you are feeling is meant for you. You get to have all of this "I'm pregnant" goodness.

Claiming this pregnancy as being meant for you isn't just about acknowledging the presence of this good fortune. It will also serve as a shield against the fear and doubt that will unquestionably cross your path as you live the next forty-ish weeks. Women who believe the good in their lives was meant for them move with a more confident stride, are more resilient, and show up to challenges with a steadier hand. It's not about entitlement or hubris, but rather a deep and abiding trust. While your fertility journey may have shaken your trust in many things, the appearance of the two lines is a clear invitation to begin repairing it. Just notice how the words *"This was meant for me"* feel in your body. Even if you have to say the phrase a few times for the words to register, there is an unmistakable resonance. A truth. Even some peace.

Resist the temptation to overanalyze the meaning of "This was meant for me." Do yourself and this baby a favor and just accept it as truth. In the glow of this moment, you get to do just that!

As I mentioned earlier, I have more to say about embracing the good in your life, as I suspect that's something you sometimes struggle with (wink wink), so don't worry. Smart cookies will tuck a shortened version of my statement of faith in their back pocket in case of mindset emergencies: *This was meant for me.*

THIS PREGNANCY IS A DANCE WITH YOUR BABY

In the spirit of "This was meant for me," and to help you keep the fears about what lies ahead at bay, I want to give you a kinder, gentler, and decidedly softer way to see this time in your life. This pregnancy is a dance that you will do with this baby. You are partners in this process. The two of you are joined in a bond that you've only shared with one other person—your own mom! This is unique, special, and sacred. You will be moving together through this time, making interdependent moves—interestingly, with your baby as the lead.

Now, that last part may have you thinking, "Huh?" But it's

true. You must remember that this baby has their own soul, their own knowing, their own personality, and their own intelligence. This child chose to be here with you, in this moment! Waltzing with the metaphor, this baby asked you to dance. You have no idea what turns you will take or exactly how you will glide across the floor, but one thing is for sure: you will be doing it together. It's not just you, Mama, and frankly, it's not all about you. This pregnancy is something you do together. When you combine "This was meant for me" with "We are doing this together," you can breathe.

I also want to underscore an incredibly important point that is often lost in the initial joy and craziness of finding out you are pregnant: you have everything you need to handle whatever shows up in the coming months inside of you. You've seen the dragon, Mama! Your fertility journey has prepared you for this moment. All the ups, downs, and uncertainty you endured showed you aspects of yourself you probably had no idea existed. You get to call upon all that rich awareness now. Your journey was preparation. While indeed the circumstances are different and some would argue that the stakes are higher, I am willing to bet that deep down, you know there are a wealth of resources within you that you can tap into at any time to carry you through. For sure the terrain has changed... *but so have you.*

KATHY DANCED WITH HER BABY ALL THE WAY TO MAMA TOWN

To give you an example of what embracing the dream, doing the dance with your baby, and knowing that you have everything within you right now to face this pregnancy with confidence, joy, and peace looks like, I want to share the story of my beloved client Dr. Kathy. As both an attorney and practicing physician, Kathy was used to working hard, setting goals, and earning what she wanted, but her fertility journey threw a massive monkey wrench in the otherwise neat and tidy program of her life. Facing low ovarian reserve and having lived through miscarriage and treatment failures, Kathy felt like the odds seemed stacked against her. But, on the eve of starting a three-cycle embryo banking series, she thumbed her nose at the statistics and found out she was pregnant naturally. (Seriously—she found out she was pregnant days before starting the process.)

As excited and blown away as she was, her immediate fear was that something terrible would happen again. A critical aspect of the coaching I gave her was about *embracing this miracle*. She had to take a step back, let go of how things were "supposed to go," and receive this gift. I coached her to trust herself and this baby, so they could do this dance together knowing that everything she had been through on her fertility journey had prepared her for this.

When Kathy started to apply these concepts to her pregnancy, she was able to reduce her anxiety and allow herself to enjoy this incredible surprise blessing through every stage of her pregnancy. When she got scared, she went back to the principle that her son chose to be with her in a very unexpected way—*this was meant for her*.

I will never forget the day that Kathy sent me pictures of her newborn son. Vibrant, precious, and miraculous. He was indeed meant for her. If you want to learn more about Kathy's story, listen to her tell it in her own words in this interview on my YouTube channel: https://youtu.be/W-l7dfCT9-I.

PUT AN END TO "NOW WHAT?"

Coming back to the question—"I'm pregnant, OMG, now what?"—that's undoubtedly nagging at you in the background as you read this, I'm going to invite you to answer in an unexpected way: with a promise. Most of the time, when our fear presents us with questions, we tend to answer with sheepish justifications or flimsy "I don't know"s. Having had the grit and tenacity to make it to this place in your fertility journey, you and this baby deserve better than that. You deserve the kind of peace and certainty *only you* can create with a clear and bold statement. With that said, here's an exercise: **Your Pregnancy Promise.**

On a sheet of paper or on a page in your pregnancy journal (if you don't already have one, I strongly suggest you get one— you'll want to be a good historian of this time in your life), write down a single promise that you make to yourself and this baby. Simplicity is key, so make it a single sentence. The first time you realize the two of you are in the same place at the same time, *here and now*, is something that happens once. Memorialize it with a promise. This can be anything you choose. An example of this could be:

- I promise to focus on love.
- I promise to surround you with joy and peace.
- I promise to protect our peace.
- I promise to keep my heart open and to follow your lead.
- I promise to nourish the both of us with healthy food, healthy people, and faith.

Let this one promise reflect who you are, what you value, and what you aspire to be as you live this time in your life. When you finish writing out your promise, take a moment to close your eyes and let the words take hold in your mind. Feel the power in the simple statement you have written. Decide that you will come back to it often to stay grounded and focused.

With this promise, you are making a commitment to yourself and to your baby from this moment on. Whether you just found out you are pregnant or are further along in your pregnancy, now is the perfect time to decide how you choose to show up and exactly "who" you will be. Not only will this serve as your foundation for this pregnancy, but it will also keep you anchored to truth when the temptations of fear, doubt, or negativity come creeping, as we know they undoubtedly will.

You are exactly where you are meant to be, Mama. Embrace it. Enjoy it. Make yourself a promise.

Next, I will be sharing some powerful ideas about how you will navigate the early weeks of your pregnancy—fearlessly.

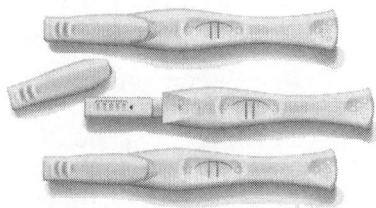

Chapter 3

I'm Pregnant... and Kinda Scared

W hile there's no question that you momentarily basked in the excitement of seeing those two lines, I am sure that, despite my best efforts in the last chapter, your mind was racing to get out of that warm and fuzzy moment so you could just get down to the proverbial brass tacks of:

Seriously! I want to have a scan pronto so I can see with my own two eyes that this baby is really in there. I want every reassurance possible that they are going to stay for good! I want to know THIS is it! Could there be a twenty-four-hour prenatal clinic?

I understand the impulse, sister. I get what it's like to be riding over rainbows on the back of a unicorn one minute and to be in abject terror that the rug is going to be pulled out from underneath you the next. I also know that allowing that fear-based urgency to run the show is a mistake. It's one thing to be excited; it's another to be fearful and grasping at anything to quell the rumblings of your Saboteurs. And, truth be told, you know the difference.

YES, I'M EXCITED... BUT WILL IT STICK?

The first days and weeks of your pregnancy, especially as a woman who struggled with fertility for some time, may be some of the most challenging. You are waiting to have your pregnancy confirmed by a blood test. You are waiting to find out your level of pregnancy hormone—is it healthy, is it doubling? It seems like, for every answer, there are only more (increasingly anxiety-fueled) questions.

What's unique to women on this journey is that we are so used to being monitored like science experiments that the time between each test or poke or prod can seem like an eternity. This creates within us a funny dependency on constant monitoring and near-instant results. After the initial blood tests, it may be up to a couple of weeks before you have your first scan... *Eeeeeek!* You might be rightfully asking yourself, *How the hell am I going to fill the time?! I don't know what to do with myself!* I am sure that more than a few of you reading this seriously considered the possibility of getting your hands on an ultrasound machine and doing some DIY ultrasounds, straight-up *I Love Lucy* style. Stop it! Don't even think about it. There are some much wiser and more well-advised things you can do to not just "deal" with the anxiety but thrive in the face of it.

THE TRUTH ABOUT WHAT MAKES EARLY PREGNANCY "SCARY"

One of the primary culprits making the early days of pregnancy so agonizing is our tendency, in the face of uncertainty, to try to assuage our fears by looking for analogous situations from the past or swinging to the polar opposite, "future-tripping." What makes this understandable but deeply flawed approach problematic is that it robs us of the miracle that is unfolding in the now. We can't see the miracle of this moment when we are reliving the past or trying to Nostradamus our way through the future.

If you find yourself sandwiched between the past and future, you've got to keep something important in mind: they are both figments of our imagination! I know you may be thinking: "What are you talking about, Rosanne? I lived my past. I was there! How am I making it up?!" Well, memory science proves that our memories are not just neutral parties simply cataloging the events of our lives. Our memories are shaded by our biases and our emotions, as well as by cultural, societal, or religious influences. We, in essence, remember things as we choose to remember them (consciously or unconsciously). We are not purely neutral, objective observers.

As a prosecutor, I witnessed this firsthand in the courtroom. You could have ten people witness the same incident but come up with ten different descriptions of events. Yes, there would be similarities, and some events might match up squarely, but each person would see things differently, sometimes markedly so. So, once we can acknowledge that we're not objective observers, it's not surprising to accept that, when it comes to our past, at some level, we are kind of making it up. We see things through the lens of our experience—not necessarily as they objectively are.

A well-documented coping mechanism we use as humans is to look for patterns to create a sense of certainty. This is how we assess whether something newly presented is friend or foe. That means that if there is anything in our present that looks at all like our past, we will immediately associate the two and (at least temporarily) assume they are the same—good or bad. We jump to the conclusion that if what's in the present looks at all like the past, *it must be history repeating itself.* That is rarely the case. A prime example of this is the way we analyze the symptoms we have leading up to a pregnancy test. If we have symptoms of PMS coming on, it *must* mean we aren't pregnant because when we've felt those symptoms in the past, our test was negative. However, in my experience, that leap in logic is wrong as often as it is right! Early pregnancy symptoms and PMS have a lot in common. I've talked many a woman off the proverbial ledge who was 100% convinced her test would be negative, only to find out she was wrong! This has proven true even for women who have had pregnancies in the past and were convinced they'd "know" if they were pregnant. This is exactly why mining the past for some semblance of "certainty" in the present is so dangerous. We quite literally rob ourselves of the objectivity that can keep us steady and calm in the present.

What if, while similar, this new situation in your life is actually nothing like your past? What opportunities and nuances do you completely miss because you automatically assume that the two situations are identical? Taking the time to consider these questions can save you a good deal of grief, Mama. Think about what you are thinking about before you jump to any conclusions based on the past.

The same is true when we go down the road of trying to predict the future. Indeed, our level of conjecture may be a bit higher because we have not yet experienced the events, but we use the same mechanism of imagination to fill in the blanks and try to extrapolate possible outcomes. It's true that your experience can help you make educated guesses about how events may unfold, but they are guesses, nonetheless.

The fear that often counterbalances our joy (at best) or steals it (at worst) in the early days of pregnancy is the very real fact that we have no idea what's going on "in there." Yes, we have blood tests that will tell us our human chorionic gonadotropin (hCG) is going up appropriately, consistent with healthy pregnancy. We may or may not have pregnancy symptoms that strongly suggest our pregnancies are progressing. But until we have our first scans, we don't really know what's up.

As women who have struggled to get to this place in our lives, our immediate concern, particularly if we have experienced the loss of pregnancy in the past, is whether this pregnancy will go the distance and result in a healthy, happy baby. This is not unreasonable and is most certainly our Mama Bear energy kicking in (we will talk more about this later), but the "edge" this feeling has with us is very different from that of a woman who didn't struggle with fertility. It's not better or worse; it's just different. It can feel like the stakes are higher—and indeed, for us, let's be honest, they are.

THE FEAR OF EARLY PREGNANCY LOSS

It is for the reasons above that, before we go any further, I want to address the subject of loss in two distinct ways, the second being a perspective you might not expect. I know you might feel a little frightened by or superstitious about the subject of loss, but I'm not raising it here to scare you. If I haven't made myself abundantly clear, let me do so now: everything I am trying to do in this book is about empowering you. I want to help you understand (from experience—my own and that of my clients) what is probably happening for you and how to approach it so you aren't weaponless when the haranguing, gravelly voice of loss-related "what if"s shows up. *And it will.* This isn't fear porn; it's part of being Fearless.

(If reading this section right now doesn't feel great, just dog-ear the page and come back to it when you are ready.)

First, whether you've had loss in the past or you haven't but are concerned it could show up somewhere in the future (before you enter the twelve-week "safe zone"), I want you to know you aren't crazy or even particularly neurotic. Pregnancy loss happens. It happens to women of all ages, regardless of whether the pregnancy was natural or the result of treatment. It happens for reasons we know and those that we don't. It sucks. It's heartbreaking. It can render you temporarily helpless.

The subject of loss is particularly scary for women on the other side of our fertility journeys because we think to ourselves, "I'm pregnant! Woo-hoo! I finally got my ticket off this fertility crazy train. The nightmare is over." The thought of ever having to step back into a life of endless doctor's appointments, supplements, medication, and procedures and risk being hurt again is about as enticing as a return to Alcatraz mere hours after making a harrowing escape and tasting the sweet nectar of freedom. There's a part of us that wonders how much more we can take and if we can keep going.

But the fear isn't just rooted in our stamina; it's a fear of lamenting what could have been, a fear of the high hopes for *this baby* being taken away, of having to deal with questions from those around us, and of the unsolicited pitying looks we might get. The burden of emotional pain *we imagine* dwarfs any physical pain we might endure. The fear of that kind of grief is enough to send anyone into the magnetic grip of anxiety.

I will be sharing many different tools in this book to address the various ways that fear can come up—because it has a multitude of faces. No matter how they may cloak themselves, your darkest fears during this pregnancy all lead back to what we are talking about here. With what I give you in this book, you will be well-equipped.

For the time being, the smartest thing you can do is acknowledge that loss happens. There are no guarantees in this life, so acknowledge the possibility. But let me be clear:

acknowledging the possibility is not the same as *focusing on it* and allowing it to suck the joy out of your pregnancy. Acknowledge it, but as a real—but remote—possibility. Even if you have had losses in the past, review what I shared earlier: the past does not predict the future. Acknowledge the fear, then set your focus on *this pregnancy* and the joyous possibilities that lie ahead. Supported by the tools that I will be giving you in this book, just know that you have everything inside of you *right now* that you may need to face anything that lies ahead with courage and resilience.

COULD PAST LOSSES ACTUALLY BE GAINS?

In order to truly appreciate the second approach to loss that I am sharing with you here—not just so that you can receive this idea with the good intent that it is given, but so that you can immediately use it to calm your nerves—we must agree on one critical point: it is 100% possible for two things to be true at the same time. Put another way, two seeming opposites can coexist. For example, you can be both happy for someone *and* jealous of them at the same time. I hear women on this journey say that all the time: "I am so happy for my pregnant sister-in-law, but at the same time, as embarrassed as I am to admit it, I'm jealous."

We are complex beings, capable of processing complicated and seemingly juxtaposed emotions. We all have this ability within us, but we are often urged to "pick a side" when it comes to our emotions. We are rushed into categorizing them conveniently so that others can more easily comprehend what we are going through. Or, even worse, we are shamed for being able to see the silver lining in tough situations and are thereby slapped with the obnoxious label of "toxic positivity." The irony is that the *real* toxicity is the refusal to acknowledge that, in nature, everything has an opposite: in/out, up/down, dark/light, high/low, "good"/"bad," lack/abundance, love/hate... you get the picture. What at the outset might look like misery could be a blessing in disguise.

It is upon the premise that two things can be true at the same time that I want to invite you to consider a tenet that I live by and teach my ladies: *see your "losses" as gains.* I know part of you may gasp at what I just said, particularly in the context of pregnancy loss, but hear me out. Having lived through pregnancy loss myself and having coached countless women through it, as a survivor and as an observer, I know for a fact that, as painful physically and emotionally as a loss may be, what lies on the other side unquestionably moves you closer to your healthy, happy baby.

(I know this may be hard to accept, but stick with me—remember, you are reading this book because you want to live your pregnancy in peace and joy. That's what I'm helping you do!)

We don't always know why losses occur, as they can happen at any time in otherwise perfectly healthy pregnancies. Even when there is an "explanation," a diagnosis alone provides little solace. What does foster resilience and provide comfort and direction is the fact that Mother Nature is undeniably wise. All one must do is look around our natural world to see that this is true. For every seeming tragedy, she comes through with something miraculous. Our bodies' innate abilities to heal, even when "science" has written us off for dead, is a readily accessible testimony to this fact. We all know someone who "shouldn't have survived" but did. We've also heard the stories of women who had a less than 1% chance of getting pregnant by any means—*and did.* My ladies do exactly that on the regular!

Seeing losses as gains is about embracing the idea that Nature is benevolent, even if we don't understand her methods or her reasoning. Just as she will miraculously save a mama's life when the odds are against it or make a miracle pregnancy possible, she will also intervene when something is not right and our babies are not healthy.

Our science as human beings is extremely limited, and we've barely scratched the surface of the known Universe. I've even heard it said that honest scientists will admit that, when it comes to all that could be known about the Universe, we know about .005% of what is "out there." This is a humbling notion and an invitation to consider that there are explanations for circumstances beyond our current level of comprehension. When we take that into account and make the conscious decision to see nature as good, then we open our minds and hearts to the idea that yes, a loss is extremely painful, *and* loss happens for the highest good—not as punishment or revenge for some past "wrong." Remember, two things can be true at the same time.

Seeing losses as gains is not an attempt to bypass the very real pain we experience. Rather, it is a much-needed higher consciousness counterbalance to the egoic, victimhood-laden notion that anything "negative" that happens in our lives is both inherently evil and permanent. In presenting you with this idea, I am not suggesting that seeing losses as gains is an instant panacea for your pain. Instead, let this idea be a light that guides you through the darkness. I know that when I miscarried the pregnancy I had before my pregnancy with Asher, this belief kept me steady in the deepest moments of my anger, despair, and heartbreak.

There is always something good coming for you, Mama. That doesn't mean there won't be challenges, but remember that, whether we can see it in the moment or not, the Universe is always conspiring in our favor, even when there appears to be a temporary roadblock. I realize that you may not immediately onboard the idea of seeing losses as gains, but I encourage you to, at the very least, tuck this idea into your back pocket for safekeeping.

I know that, for some, the fear of loss isn't necessarily around early pregnancy. It is possible that your darkest fear is that later in your pregnancy, when your heart is even more vulnerable, you will find out something is "wrong." I will address that later in chapter 8. Let your heart be at peace now, Mama, knowing that this child showed up in your life for a reason. Breathe and let's take the tempo back up again. Remember, regardless of what your fears may be whispering to you, *You. Are. Pregnant.*

YOU MADE IT: LET THAT SINK IN... REALLY

Now that we have dealt with that elephant in the room, I think it's time to remind you of something critically important: *YOU MADE IT, MAMA!*

Because you dared to be the woman who refused to give up...

Because you stayed your course, refused to be thwarted by "scary" statistics, were open to getting the side-eye from friends, family, medicine, and any other naysayers...

...you are pregnant!

There's so much to be celebrating about being in this place, but, at the core, the "win" isn't found in the fact that you're finally having the baby you dreamed of. Yes, it's glorious that your baby has made their appearance, but what I want to help you acknowledge is who you've become. It is no small feat to be the woman who trusts herself and her vision despite the barking jackals of negativity all around.

I know your tendency is to say, "That's just what I do" and blow this accomplishment off, but I urge you not to do that. *We build trust in ourselves when we focus on the evidence in our lives that demonstrates we are trustworthy.* You followed through on your dream. That means you can trust yourself to "do what it takes."

This information is priceless when we consider the automatic negative thoughts that pop up almost constantly. Focusing on the things we've done to follow through and live our dream builds our level of credibility with the most important audience of all: ourselves.

For this reason, I am going to give you an exercise that, if you take the time to do it—and I mean do it *now*—will support your peace and resilience throughout your entire pregnancy and, ultimately, your life. Bold claim, I know, but when you do it, you will understand why I stand by it.

I call this the **Woman, You Did Good Letter**, and it's your chance to connect with the truth about you and who you really are. Here goes:

- Grab something to write on and something to write with. I strongly encourage you to handwrite this so we can slow your thought process down and activate a different part of your brain.
- Find a peaceful place where you can write uninterrupted for a minimum of fifteen minutes.
- Decide that, for that solid fifteen minutes, you will focus on this exercise and this exercise alone.
- Set a timer on your phone for fifteen minutes.
- Write a letter of appreciation to *yourself* for being the woman who dared to be tenacious, courageous, and fully committed to her dream of being a mom, in the face of naysayers, skeptics, and what others may have deemed "insane" odds.
- Hold nothing back in this letter. Be kind and generous, and give yourself the gift of well-deserved (and seldom-received) kudos. Let this letter be a love letter of sorts to your highest, most Fearless self—the woman you are most proud of being.
- Include specific examples of how you stood your ground and dared to believe, and how it felt to (at times) be the "last woman on the dance floor."

- Be a good steward of your personal history here, as it will serve as an indispensable reminder in the face of uncertainty that, indeed, you can trust yourself to go the distance. You can trust *you!*
- When you are done with the fifteen minutes, if you feel like writing more, feel free to do so. Lavish yourself with well-deserved love. If you are done at fifteen minutes, great!
- Review what you wrote once. Then, read it to yourself *out loud*. Yes, out loud. This is critical because we hear the voices of our Saboteurs almost constantly as we move through the day. Let them hear some long-overdue counterfacts. Notice how it feels to hear the words you read about yourself.
- Put this tribute to yourself in a place where you can find it easily. If you included it in your journal, mark the page so that you can find it quickly when you are having a "moment" and need a powerful reminder of how awesome and badass you are.
- Make a promise to yourself that you won't forget what it felt like to hear this truth.

TOOLS FOR STAYING CALM AND CONFIDENT

Now that you have facts and powerful reminders of how trust-worthy and awesome you really are, let's add to the mix some critically important tools and ideas for keeping you feeling peace, calm, and confidence in the early days and weeks of your pregnancy. One of the things I hear about all the time (and have experienced myself) is the odd mix of anxiety and excitement we wrestle with at the beginning of our "beat-the-odds" preg-nancy. When the road to pregnancy wasn't easy and it seemed like you'd never get to this place, it can be hard to believe it's happening, and it can feel too good to be true. As much as you are excited to see your baby on that black-and-white ultrasound screen, there's likely a tiny voice in the back of your mind freaking you out that the ultrasound tech won't see anything or that she'll tell you that there's something wrong with what she does see. The anticipation is nerve-racking.

What's heartbreaking about this thought pattern is that, left unchecked, it will rob you of the moments when you thought you'd be happiest. Seriously, you were dying to get to this point, but now you find yourself agonizing over whether what you will see is sufficient?! Let's stop that insanity right now with what I call the **Pre-Scan Calming Ritual**.

The "ritual" I describe here is something that you can use prior to any prenatal scan, checkup, blood test, or screening that causes you to feel anxious. It is simple and quick:

- Find a quiet place to sit—whether in your clinic or the hospital or even in your car before walking into your appointment—for just one minute.
- While seated, close your eyes and imagine a soft, beautiful ball of pink light forming around you, creating a protective space between you and the world outside.
- In this ball of pink light, there is nothing but peace, connection to your baby, and gratitude that you are even in the position to have a prenatal appointment.
- With this pink light all around you, there is nothing but the presence of GUS (God/Universe/Source)— and you allow yourself to feel it all around. You feel safe and loved.
- Take three deep, slow inhales and exhales, then repeat this statement: *Being a mom was meant for me. The highest good is coming for me and my baby. I trust myself; I trust my body; I trust this baby.*
- Repeat the last step twice!

The point of this exercise is to get you out of your head and back into your body with a clear and calm statement of truth and trust. Just notice how you feel when you do it. Dare I say, it's magic.

This same ritual of love and trust can be used during any of the milestone or "goalpost" type appointments we have in the early days and weeks of pregnancy, such as the scan for a heart-beat, seeing that the baby is continuing to grow at a healthy rate, and getting to the "safety" of twelve weeks.

IS IT SAFE TO POOP, AND AM I SICK ENOUGH?

For us as women who struggled with fertility, each appointment often tends to be a cliffhanger to the next, as we are seeking almost constant reassurance that our baby is okay. While it's good to acknowledge that, at least in part, this comes from Mama Bear energy (again, I will say more about that later), the fact remains that being on the "other side" of our journey can feel like being in wild, uncharted territory. We need as much reassurance as we can get, and, interestingly enough, we might need such reassurance every time we go to the bathroom.

What?! Yes. It's true.

Who knew that the seemingly innocuous act of going to the bathroom could send otherwise reasonable women into a tail-spin? It's what I refer to as being on Pee Patrol. This is when you are so scared of having the pregnancy rug pulled out from underneath you that you are quite literally terrified to pee because you're afraid that you will see blood. When you are that scared, blood automatically = miscarriage, *even though that's not always what it means.* If I had a dime for every time a woman told me she was afraid to pee, I'd be writing this book from my beach house in St. Barths. I've even had women share that they were terrified of pooping because they were afraid that if there was any straining, their baby would come out!

Think about that. Many of us are at such a level of distrust of our bodies, ourselves, and the Universe that we are afraid of normal, healthy bodily functions that you want to engage in daily!

As seemingly ridiculous as this may sound, it is quite revealing about the fear we create for ourselves on this journey. This time in our lives could be so full of joy if we only allowed it to be. While it is true that nobody wants to have a miscarriage, and I have already acknowledged the very real pain of it, when we get to the point where we can't use the bathroom without fear, we must admit there's a problem.

This same brand of fear shows itself in another way that women torture themselves on this journey, which is what I call the "Am I Sick Enough?" game. In the first days and weeks of pregnancy, truth be told, if we aren't worried about seeing blood when we pee, we are agonizing over whether we feel *pregnant enough*. We take the symptom-spotting we did *before* we found out we were pregnant to the next hysterical level. If we aren't doubled over with nausea with painful breasts or lethargy, we start freaking out that our pregnancy symptoms are waning and end up driving our anxiety to its next peak. When we add the "Am I Sick Enough?" Game to Pee Patrol, it's a wonder that we don't collapse under the weight of our own anxiety—and the sad part is, some do.

INTEGRITY, PRESENCE, AND A PRAYER

The question becomes how we can thoughtfully and intentionally navigate the real concerns we might have with the often-trumped-up terror that our Saboteurs create. Let me give you three powerful solutions.

First, I want you to think back to the days before you were pregnant. Remember how you said you'd be when you finally got pregnant? Chances are, you told yourself that when you got "there" you would be so happy and grateful that nothing could bring you down. Yeah, be *that* woman. I'm serious. We tend to completely forget the promises we made ourselves when times were tough. Be a woman of integrity. With that being said, here's your first tool in this section: **Be the Woman You Said You'd Be.** Instead of cowering in the presence of fear, remember the image you had created in your mind of bliss, confidence, and gratitude. The woman you imagined is still in there. She's just waiting for you to call her up onstage.

Your next tool is **Stay Present.** When I say "stay present," I mean stay in this moment, *now*. As I described in detail earlier in this chapter, our tendency when frightened is to revert to the past or start using our imagination unwisely about the future. The scenarios of doom, gloom, and misery are all too readily available in either direction, so stay in the now.

When you think about it, unless something horrendous is immediately befalling you *now*, the truth is that you are safe. In this moment, you are pregnant, your baby is growing, and all is well. Let the past be the past. The past has nothing to do with what's true today. The same idea is true about any fear-based machinations you might be entertaining about the future. The past and future live solely in your imagination. Press pause on your imagination—you don't need it right now. Your pregnant present is enough.

The simplest and quickest way to yank yourself out of the past or future is to ask yourself, "What am I feeling in my body now?" Maybe you just sipped some tea and can feel the warm liquid in your mouth. Perhaps you can feel yourself sitting in your chair or on your sofa. Maybe you are outside and can feel the warmth of the sun on your face. Wherever you are, ask the question. It will immediately bring you back to the here and now. When you do it, you will begin to see how far you have drifted off into the past or future. It's kind of crazy when you experience the shift between the past or future and the now. Stay present and in peace, Mama.

Another tool that I will share here is a prayer that I call **It's You and I, Little One**. If the word "pray" doesn't work for you, feel free to call this a "conversation" instead.

This prayer has no denomination and is intended to be a celebration of the innate connection with your child. My ladies find it super helpful, particularly when they struggle with feeling connected to something they can't yet see. We will discuss faith later in this book because it is such an integral aspect of confidence, peace, and joy on this journey, but for now, just focus on the simple prayer or conversation prompt I offer you here:

It's you and I, little one. Mommy loves you so much, and I am so glad you are here. I've wanted to have you for so long. There are times when I get scared, but don't let my fear be yours. We will be together.
I love you. I trust you. We are a team. Together we pray for and expect the highest good. I will be here for you… always.

This prayer is an affirmation of an expectation of the highest good, whatever that may be. It is a statement of commitment to your child and an acknowledgment that whether it is their time to make it Earthside or not, you will be there for them. It's about not making the outcome personal or taking anything about your pregnancy personally. While that last part may be hard to grasp, give yourself a chance to kick the idea around a bit. You may warm to it as you read and learn more.

ROBYN AND RUBY: A STORY FIFTEEN YEARS IN THE MAKING

To bring many of the concepts I have shared with you here into a practical context, I want to share the story of my beloved client Robyn and her miracle daughter, Ruby. When Robyn came to me, she had been on her fertility journey for nearly fifteen years. She had one beautiful miracle son who came to her with the support of IVF, and while she wanted another child, with health challenges for both her and her husband, Robyn knew that completing her family would not be "easy." But from the moment I first spoke with her, she knew she had a daughter on her heart, and that daughter's name was Ruby.

Both Robyn and her husband had grown weary after so many years of treatment, but Robyn simply could not rest until Ruby was here. During our time together, Robyn made the decision that she would try IVF again, with a protocol that was specifically tailored to her needs. We worked rigorously on her mindset, dragging out old Saboteurs and taming the stories that threatened to weaken her resolve. Those around her struggled to believe in Robyn's vision, but she insisted on moving forward on her terms.

After her last transfer, Robyn's anxiety hit a fever pitch because she believed she was getting her period. She sent me a text, convinced the cycle had failed and certain that the bleeding she saw was her period. Unconvinced that the cycle had failed, I urged her to use some of the tools that I have shared with you here. Lo and behold, despite the blood she saw, when Robyn later took a pregnancy test, *it was positive*. The positive test was then confirmed by her doctor.

Fear had temporarily distracted Robyn from the truth: having Ruby was meant for her. We could not stop screaming with joy! Robyn continued to apply the strategies that I taught her and refused to let her fear and anxiety rob her of the bliss that came as the result of baby Ruby beating the odds to get here. And, as of this writing, baby Ruby just turned nine months old.

(If you want to hear Robyn tell you this story herself, you can check out my Fearlessly Fertile podcast, episode 108, or watch our interview here: https://youtu.be/103o90AMiQ8.)

Through everything I have shared in this chapter, Mama, I

want you to know that I absolutely have compassion for the anxiety you feel in these early days of your pregnancy. I also know that compassion is nothing without active support. This is why I have spoken to you in the direct way that I have and shared active tools and strategies for quickly addressing the fears that so often come up during this very special, unique, and challenging time. There are few times when your mindset on this journey will be challenged more. Just know that, with what I have given you here, your quiver is well stocked.

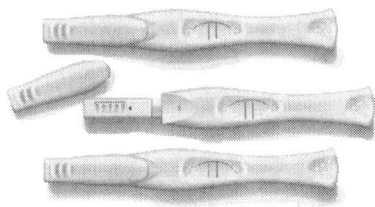

Chapter 4

Okay, This Pregnancy Thing Is Real

After the initial excitement and cray cray of early pregnancy starts to wane, there is a very interesting question that begins to creep into our minds. It's both unsettling and a bit shocking, so at first, we bat it away like an annoying fly, but it buzzes back again and again. We fear answering it because it seems weird and ungrateful. We continue to avoid it because we innately sense that it will bring up complex feelings within us that we thought would magically go away once we were pregnant. Here's the question: *"Is this all there is?"*

While you might use slightly different language to ask this question, the sentiment is the same. I know this question has crossed your mind because, once all the rushing around and the frenzy of first appointments dies down and the transition into prenatal care begins, you settle back into your life where, for the most part, everything is pretty much the same. *The only difference is that you are pregnant.*

Don't get me wrong; that is a blessed and glorious change, but we often go back to living as we always have, which drags us to this complicated question. It's like there's this massive rush of emotion and, when the dust settles, we find ourselves back in our same old lives... with a twist, in the shape of a growing bump. It can almost feel like a "hurry up and wait" situation.

I want to let you know this is normal. You aren't an ungrateful jerk or weirdo if you aren't having Hallmark movie moments every second just because you saw those two coveted lines. You are human, Mama! We create these Hollywood-worthy dramas in our minds about what life will be like the instant we are pregnant, but those dramas rarely match reality. Being surprised that your reality doesn't match what you imagined doesn't mean there's a "letdown" about being pregnant, it's just that our fantasy doesn't quite square up to reality... *unless, of course, we make the conscious decision to make it so.* But, before I show you how to do that, let's acknowledge an important truth.

WHEN YOU REALIZE PREGNANCY DIDN'T CHANGE... MUCH

The "problems" and complexities that existed prior to your pregnancy aren't just going to disappear the day you find out you are pregnant. My guess is that, as an intelligent woman, you know this, but the emotional side of you needs to hear it— otherwise, the blips of disillusionment you will undoubtedly feel (even briefly) will catch you off guard. When we have struggled to achieve something for so long and we finally get "there," a time will come when we realize that our lives are pretty much the same... just different, if that makes sense. Pregnancy doesn't suddenly permanently repair your self-esteem, worthiness, or sense of wholeness. Yes, it will give you one hell of a boost, but you will soon come to understand that this business of working on yourself isn't over. You will still argue with your partner, boundaries with family will still be violated, your coworkers will still wear you out, your friends might still let you down, you will still get speeding tickets, your wrinkles won't suddenly go away, and your care team will still do silly things.

None of this is "bad." It just serves to underscore the perils of destination thinking. If you've never heard that term before, it describes the thought process that many of us engage in when we think that everything is going to suddenly change for the better (and all our problems will be resolved) when we get to a certain level of achievement or accomplish some "thing." If the words, "I will be so happy when_____" have ever come out of your mouth, that's a prime example of destination thinking. It's the kind of thinking that can hold our joy, peace, worthiness, and confidence hostage until some arbitrary criteria is met—*and this criteria is often a moving target.* There are many athletes, celebrities, entrepreneurs, and high achievers across various disciplines who have acknowledged this phenomenon. Whether it was winning a gold medal, getting an Oscar, or making their first million dollars, shortly after the initial excitement wore off, a sense of "Is this all there is?" started creeping in. This is a direct result of destination thinking.

My guess is you understand this intellectually, but at some level, we secretly imagine that all the pain and emptiness we feel in our lives will go away with the arrival of this baby. It won't, and you certainly don't want to saddle this baby with that burden! Just know that if you find yourself in this place of "Is this all there is?", don't beat yourself up. It happens to the best of us, and you find yourself in good company.

As I said before, you are human… and pregnant. *(I threw that in there as a joyful reminder. I know you probably still get a thrill hearing it!)*

WILL YOU MAKE YOUR PREGNANCY WHAT YOU HOPED IT WOULD BE?

This phenomenon presents you with an extremely exciting and life-changing opportunity, Mama. Your pregnancy is in many ways a fork in the road—will you continue to live life as you always have, or will you truly step into being the woman you always imagined and dreamed you would be?

People look at me funny when I describe a woman's struggle with fertility as an existential crisis, but I believe it is. It certainly calls into question all our beliefs, particularly when it comes to what we think is possible for us in this life. It challenges the programming we were raised with and what we believe we are worthy of having. It may even change our perception of family entirely. That means that, when we finally get and stay pregnant, we have the chance to take all the lessons we've learned and the new awareness we have gained to consciously construct the women we choose to be in this transformational chapter in our lives. Instead of being the woman watching other women make their mom dreams come true, you are now one of them.

You get to see yourself as a woman who defied the odds.

Just take that sentence in for a moment. There is so much power in it. *(If there's part of you that resists this idea, go back and read the letter you wrote yourself in chapter 3.)* You have the chance to continue becoming the woman you said you would be when you were pregnant—which is why I presented that idea to you in the last chapter.

Seizing this opportunity to be the woman you always said you'd be when you got "here" is not just about feeling empowered; it's radically practical. You must remember—now that you are pregnant, your pregnancy is progressing, and you are well into prenatal care—that *everyone else gets to go home.* The constant monitoring tapers off, the space between your appointments gets longer, and the initial rush of excitement has calmed down among the people around you—so you are left with yourself and how you are going to navigate the next weeks and months of your pregnancy. It's exciting, sobering, and your official entry into "the club."

YOU'RE AN OFFICIAL MEMBER OF THE CLUB... BUT FEEL LIKE A WANNABE

I'm bringing your attention to the fact that you are an official member of the "Pregnant Lady Club" because I know that those of us who have spent so long on our fertility journeys have a tendency toward not really seeing ourselves in that way. In many ways, it's a crisis of identity. We've identified with being in struggle around this topic for so long that, when we get to this place, we still feel a bit like a "wannabe" or impostor. I'm here to say a loving—but firm—*stop it.* You get to step into the fact that you are a full-on pregnant lady, Mama. We thoroughly exposed the fear-based games we play in the previous chapter. What you get to do now is begin to exercise the full range of "rights and privileges" that you thought you'd have as a gloriously glowing pregnant lady! While this may seem rather obvious to the outside world, as women who strive for excellence, we tend to be super hard on ourselves. Sometimes it takes another woman, cut from the same cloth, to remind us that we made it and encourage us to give ourselves permission to embrace the miracles we manifest. If you find yourself in that place right now, let me be the first fellow Miracle Mama to say, *"Welcome to the club!"*

An important next step to consciously constructing the pregnant lady you desire to be and thereby creating the blissful, joyous, and Fearless pregnancy you've longed for is creating a clear vision for the rest of your pregnancy. We spend a great deal of time imagining what this experience would be like *before we get pregnant*, but using your imagination to support your success doesn't end there. You will want to expand that vision to include exactly how you choose to "be" during your pregnancy, and I am going to help you do that now with my **Pregnancy Visioning Exercise**.

Pull out your journal or a fresh piece of paper to write on, as well as something to write with. Now, let's begin.

- Set the timer on your phone for fifteen minutes.
- Begin writing out (in detail) the vision that you have for your pregnancy.
- If you aren't sure where to start, pick one inspiring word that you choose to have as the intention for your pregnancy. Some examples are *peace, joy, ease, fun,* and *surrender*.
- Also be sure to include how you will choose to interact with your partner, friends, family, and the members of your care team.
- What are the big *yeses* you want to say and what are your hard *nos*?
- How do you consciously choose to respond to things that scare you or stress you out? *(Perhaps you will always keep this book within reach?)*
- What measures will you put in place to be sure that you aren't overworking and that you are making self-care a priority? Don't forget, you are growing a life inside of you! It can be exhausting.
- Finally, be sure to include ways that you will consistently connect with your baby—there is no one else you will be closer to in this life, other than your own mother!

Once you have completed your written vision for your pregnancy, put it with the Woman, You Did Good Letter you wrote yourself in chapter 3. These two loving documents will remind you of what you are capable of and who you choose to be!

IT'S TIME: BUST OUT THE GOOD CHINA

Now that you have your pregnancy vision in hand, full permission to be part of the "Pregnant Lady Club" in your heart, and an awareness that you can be anything you choose to be in this life on your mind, I want to share an idea that I like to call **Bust Out the Good China**. Far too often in this life, we hold off on relishing the full deliciousness of our daily lives until there is a special day or occasion. We only Bust Out the Good China maybe once or twice a year! We don't wear the shoes, carry the bag, or put on "the dress" unless something comes up that is so out of the ordinary, such a deviation from the humdrum norm, that it "warrants" those things. Don't do that anymore, Mama! Cherish every single moment of this pregnancy by really digging in, taking the plastic cover off things, because *this is the moment*, and *these are the days*. Quit waiting to enjoy being pregnant and telling yourself you'll do the things you said you would do when you finally got here until some later date. *Now is the time!*

This is even more important when you've experienced loss. I know that your Saboteurs will try to tell you that this is reckless and will bombard you with "what if"s, but you have to ask yourself which you would regret more: feeling alive and enjoying every moment you had with your baby, or squandering this time in your life with fear. You will never have these same days again, love. You might have them with your next baby, but not this one. Each baby and pregnancy is a unique and precious gift. For the love of all things holy, enjoy that gift!

YOUR PREGNANCY SHAPES HOW YOU WILL "MOTHER"

Another Miracle Mama nugget of wisdom that I want to share with you is the perspective that what you do now and the way you choose to live your pregnancy is helping to shape how you will show up as a mom. I make no apologies for my stance that we as women who struggled with fertility have a heightened level of responsibility for being conscious during our pregnancies and in the way that we mother our miracle babies. Our path to our children was not easy, and it was a wonderful opportunity to learn, grow, and prepare. In order to be good stewards of the blessing we are given, it is incumbent upon us to keep our eyes open and our resolve strong about how we choose to show up as mothers. Your pregnancy is the perfect time to grow in the areas of your relationships, your work-life balance, how you interact with other moms, the kind of advocate you become for your child and your family, and, ultimately, how you see yourself as a woman. Stay open and focused on the idea that I introduced to you earlier about things happening *for* you, so that you can see any experience you have during your pregnancy as preparation for becoming the mom you truly desire to be for your child.

This is also a good time to say something that you might really need to hear right now—particularly if all this mom talk is becoming a bit overwhelming. For every woman, the enormity of becoming someone's mom sets in at different times. When the road to your baby was, shall we say, "bumpy," there can be a self-inflicted extra layer of questions about your worthiness and your level of preparedness for the responsibility. You know intellectually that you are just as good as the next mama, but our self-esteem does take a beating on this journey, so if you have moments of doubt, again, you are in good company. The added twist here, especially when you are having your baby "later" in life *(Seriously, who gets to decide what's "later?")* is the worry you might be feeling about being the "older" mom or that, when compared to the other moms in the pick-up line at school, you will be seen as some kind of weird, rare, slightly pitiful bird. *Rubbish!* The truth is, you've always done things differently. It's just part of who you are. This is no better or worse; it's just different. When you take all the societal pressures and norms away, there's just you and your baby. That's truly all that matters. You are well equipped for the role of mother, and your unique path to get here will inform you in so many priceless ways. Cast off the yoke of "average" and step into your version of "normal"—which is pretty darn special.

FAITH AND YOUR FEARLESS PREGNANCY

With your pregnancy starting to feel really real, I want to raise a topic with you that can have some mixed emotions around it, but that is nonetheless an integral part of a Fearless pregnancy: faith. Before you get nervous about what I'm about to say, let me reiterate that I am not here to proselytize any particular religion or belief system. I believe that faith is a personal relationship with our Higher Power. I call that power GUS (God/Universe/Source); others call it Nature, Infinite Intelligence, their Higher Self, or whatever feels good to them. The personal relationship we have with such power is often a steadying force in our lives, and it is rarely needed more than when we are trying to navigate an entirely new set of circumstances—like pregnancy.

Chances are that you have some connection to your Higher Power, and I am encouraging you to take that faith to the next level—not just because it feels great, but because, when you have ready, consistent access to this presence, you are less likely to feel alone and overwhelmed. Think about it, Mama! This kind, generous, and benevolent energy that brought this baby to you can be a wonderful resource for peace when you need it.

One of the greatest disservices we do to ourselves on this journey is acting like lone wolves, bearing the burden of finding solutions entirely on our own, when the power of the Universe is always around us. Tap into it! Take your faith to the next level. Remember that something truly magical had to happen for your precious baby to get here. It isn't just a sperm and egg coming together! There are countless times when that happens in a lab and does not result in a pregnancy.

Something truly beyond our comprehension happens when a new life is created. If you've ever seen video of the spark of light that appears at the moment of conception, you will know to the core of your being that this is true. My ladies hear me tell them repeatedly that the desire in their hearts to be a mom is there because it was meant for them. Take comfort in the fact that Infinite Intelligence smiled upon you and brought you this baby —there must be a very good reason behind it. Let that fuel your faith, and allow yourself to explore it more deeply so that in moments of fear or uncertainty, you can rely on the fact that something higher brought you this child and will always be there to help bring your highest good to fruition.

Before I share a powerful daily practice for your Fearless pregnancy, I want to give you one more idea to consider. Allow for the messiness, Mama. You've never been pregnant in this time and place before. Even if you've had a pregnancy in the past, this pregnancy is and will be different. So much about *you* is different! Not everything will be sparkles and unicorns, but that's not a bad thing. No matter what shows up, you are well equipped. Let this pregnancy unfold. Let yourself play, explore, and live it with your eyes fully open. Remember, mistakes and temporary setbacks are always for your good. Bask in the messiness and keep your eyes peeled for the gift within it.

THE FEARLESS PREGNANCY DAILY PRACTICE

I know my ladies well enough to be fully aware of the fact that you love predictability and structure, so with this daily practice designed especially for pregnancy, you will get both. I find that when we begin each day with intention and ritual, we give ourselves the benefit of the kind of certainty only we can generate. It doesn't make much sense to have to look outside of ourselves for the certainty we crave when it is always right under our noses.

This practice is meant to be done in the morning because when we start our days consciously, we set the tone and pace for the experience we will create. Don't worry, it won't take long—and I know that with varying levels of nausea and other pregnancy symptoms, there are days when it will be a challenge—but I promise, every day that you do it, you will be better for it. Here is your **Fearless Pregnancy Daily Practice**. Start each day by setting aside a few minutes to do the following (*before your feet hit the floor*):

- When you open your eyes, quietly acknowledge the gift of waking up. This is a power move because most people take getting up in the morning for granted, when it is not at all a given.
- Next, take just a moment to acknowledge your baby and the gratitude that you have for them being with you. Put your hands on your belly as you make the acknowledgment to feel even more connected. If you have a name for your baby, call them by their name!
- Then, connect to your Higher Power, asking for guidance, inspiration, and enhanced intuition. Commit to connecting with this power throughout the day. Over time, it will feel natural and effortless, and the peace you will feel is unlike anything else.

- Lastly, set your intention for the day by selecting a single word that will be your North Star for the day.

This practice can take five minutes or less, so make no excuses. Just commit to it. Write these steps down on a sticky note and put it on your nightstand so that each morning when you get up you have a quick and easy reminder. Doing this practice daily will keep you grounded, connected with your baby, and consciously creating your Fearless pregnancy experience.

WITH TWINS ON THE WAY, KRISTEN GOT FEARLESS

To give you an example of how everything that I've shared in this chapter can help you fully step into your pregnancy with ease while giving you full license and agency to be the most authentic version of yourself during this exciting time in your life, I want to share the story of my beloved client Kristen. An accomplished sales executive for one of the most well-known brands in the world, Kristen came to me after years of trying to conceive with her husband. Like me, Kristen is unashamed of her control-freaky ways, and she was deeply committed to having a child with her husband, who happens to be just a few years younger than her. The pressure was on!

After trying repeatedly with Kristen's own eggs, Kristen and her husband decided to accept a gift of eggs donated by another woman. They were positively thrilled and were grateful for the opportunity. Kristen got pregnant after her very first donor transfer but unfortunately miscarried soon thereafter. In preparing her for her next transfer, we focused our work on keeping her "present" and focused on motherhood being a journey, not a destination. When Kristen went for her second transfer, I coached her to switch her focus to trusting herself, her body, and the desire to be a mom. In less than fourteen days from her transfer, Kristen found out that she was pregnant again—this time with her dream pregnancy, *twins!*

As ecstatic as Kristen was, she found herself struggling to wrap her head around the enormity of the gift she had received. Once the initial rush of excitement had died down from this massive win, she also realized that she had to start working on how she was going to make it through forty weeks of pregnancy without driving herself and her husband crazy with anxiety. The pain of her recent loss kept trying to distract her from her twins.

Kristen and I worked closely on helping her allow herself to finally be a member of the "Pregnant Lady Club." I gave her assignments to go purchase her babies' clothes, buy the stroller of her dreams, and, most importantly, splurge on the bougie diaper bag she had been salivating over. The goal was to have her fully embrace this blessing and see herself as the woman worthy of such an incredible gift. By deepening her faith (as I have instructed you to do in this chapter) and allowing herself to Bust Out the Good China and be the pregnant lady she daydreamed of being, as of this writing, my beloved Kristen is within weeks of meeting her twins.

The biggest lesson I want you to take from what I have shared here is to allow yourself to fully step into the blessing of this pregnancy. Hold nothing back. Refuse to live in fear. Understand that the more joy, love, and excitement you surround this baby with, the better! You've earned your right to be here, Mama. Let this pregnancy get really real.

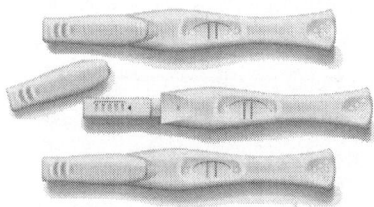

Chapter 5

Receiving: The Secret to Pregnancy Bliss

I n the years that I have been mentoring women to fertility success, one of the most consistently challenging topics my clients and I take on is receiving. What's particularly interesting about this topic is that it becomes more nuanced and more urgent to reinforce once you are pregnant. Getting my lovably high-achieving, independent, service-oriented, and often stubborn ladies to receive is like trying to pull alligator teeth at ninety-five miles an hour.

Despite such peril, I vehemently persist in teaching the power of receiving once my ladies are pregnant. (My ladies hear me say it all the time: *"Conceiving is all about receiving!"*) I believe women of the ilk that I serve struggle with this topic so much because of the "baggage" that comes along with the notion of receiving. That only gets ramped up when you receive in a *big* way, such as this pregnancy. There is a tendency to want to shrink back from receiving because we feel greedy for wanting more than this miracle pregnancy. Because I want you to have the most joyful, confident, and Fearless pregnancy ever, we will begin to unpack that load of crap here.

WHAT EXACTLY IS "RECEIVING?"

The lawyer in me demands that we define exactly what I mean when I say *receive* or *receiving*. I define *receiving* as the ability to accept love, time, money, gifts, favors, attention, support, blessings, acts of kindness, compliments, privileges, and priority without shame, guilt, condition, or the requirement of immediate and equal reciprocity. Put another way, receiving is about allowing yourself to have good in your life just because you are you. It's a celebration of your inherent value and worth as a human being without the arbitrary human construct of having to "work" for it. *Can you see why the concept of allowing yourself to receive is so powerful?* It is laden with the foundational truths that you are enough and there is enough to go around, and it is laced with unconditional love.

Take a moment to notice how your body feels when you read this definition of receiving. Do you feel resistance? Does it feel like truth, even if it's new? Does it resonate? Just notice—your answer is quite revealing about the level to which you currently allow yourself to receive. No judgment, just be aware.

If you feel any resistance to the idea of receiving in the way that I defined it here, you certainly aren't alone. I fought it at first, too, until I realized the villainous manipulation behind my resistance—did I "earn" what I received? The idea that you can only receive once you've "earned it" is a made-up concept perpetuated by those who stand to gain (often disproportion-ately) from our toil and misunderstanding of our divine nature. And what does "earning it" even mean? Who decides when you have "earned it"?

The concept of "earning it," particularly in the context of matters of the heart—such as your desire to be a mom—simply doesn't fit. "Earning it" is an idea that is more aptly applied to money, goods, and services. It implies a meritorious hierarchy that, when applied to love and your baby, just sounds gross and, frankly, inhuman. Yet, somewhere along the line, we picked up and onboarded the idea that in order to be loved or to be moth-ers, we have to "earn" those things. I've asked my ladies what "earning it" means, and many (at least, those who haven't gone through my coaching yet) describe a scenario that equals over-giving and scrounging. Not. Healthy. This is why I am proposing a definition of receiving that presupposes that you've already earned the love and baby you desire, just by being you. You were born worthy of the good you desire! There is no "earning" required. Even a cursory study of the world's sacred texts will demonstrate that receiving does not require one to give to star-vation in order to "earn" or be worthy.

If you find yourself questioning this idea, then next time someone tries to make you "wrong" for having what you desire or taking a stand for your worth, simply ask yourself, "What scares them about me receiving?" Chances are that the person who gripes about you receiving or taking a stand for your worth and value loses leverage over you. They lose an element of control over you, and they fear you moving past them in some way. When your needs are met, you don't "need" that person anymore.

Be mindful of those in your life who require you to "earn" in order to receive in matters of the heart; they rarely tend to be cheerful and generous givers. You may see this toxic pattern in friends, family, coworkers, employers, and perhaps even in your relationship. The good news is that when you accept the idea of receiving that I am presenting here, you can set a wonderful new example for those around you. They might not "get" it, but they may be inspired by it.

HEY, PREGNANT LADY: IT'S OKAY TO HAVE NEEDS!

Let's direct this concept of receiving back to your miracle pregnancy. Stated plainly, *woman, you have a precious life growing inside you. It's okay to have needs!* There's so much going on inside of you physically, mentally, and spiritually that it makes perfect sense that you will need and desire more. The trick here will be to allow yourself to receive it.

I know my ladies well enough to understand that asking for what you want or for the help you need is difficult. We'd rather run ourselves to the brink of cross-eyed exhaustion than wave the white flag. We tend to see asking for help as weak. While we would never put that label on anyone around us, we apply it to ourselves—liberally. On top of seeing receiving as weak, we also tend to see it as vulnerable due to the perceived quid pro quo that our upbringing and social conditioning tend to build around it. I've worked with women on six of seven continents, and I've found that, regardless of our culture or religion, it seems that, somewhere along the way, someone told us as women (this is dramatically less prevalent in men) that receiving is risky due to emotional intimacy that it might create. *The oppressive mask of perfection and invulnerability will be torn off to reveal we are (eek!) human!*

Interestingly enough, we may also carry a bit of fear around becoming too "demanding." We fear rejection by those around us for being a "burden." So instead of giving those around us the benefit of the doubt by asking for the support we desire, we suck it up, burn out, and get bitter. The time to be smart about receiving is now, Mama. The drama we create around receiving has got to stop. Not only does it keep you in a heightened level of stress, which is the last thing you need when pregnant with a miracle, but it unnecessarily creates distance between you and the ones you love, and it perpetuates a pattern that you don't want to carry into motherhood: martyrdom.

YOUR MIRACLE BABY DOESN'T REQUIRE YOU TO BE A MARTYR

While, for the most part, we have traded the starched dresses and pearl-bedecked perfection of the June Cleaver, *Leave It to Beaver* ideal of motherhood for messy buns and yoga-pant awesomeness, there remains an expectation that we as mothers must be and do everything for our children. If we don't work fifty-plus-hour weeks and make all our children's organic baby food by hand, show up to playdates with high energy and clever conversation while planning over-the-top birthday parties, and get back to our pre-baby weight in the blink of an eye, somehow, we miss the mark of Instagrammable perfection!

While you may think you are immune to this unspoken (but blatantly obvious) pressure, think again. I am privy to conversations with women across the globe who get to this point on their fertility journeys and suddenly feel the heightened pressure and obligation that *they* must do everything to the epitome of perfection because they fought so long and hard to get "here." Having watched Miracle Mamas take themselves and their families to the brink of crisis because of this Saboteur story, let me disabuse you of it here and now: *say no to martyrdom*. Reject the idea that you must "do it all by yourself" immediately. Why? Because that is a virtual guarantee that you will get disillusioned with, exhausted by, and resentful of this family you worked so hard for.

I know that in the beginning of our pregnancies we are

flooded with romantic notions of what we desire to be as moms, but a great deal of that is fueled by patterns from the past—we believe that if our mothers did it "that way," so must we—but that couldn't be further from the truth. Decades, education, life experience, and quality of life separate your mother's experience from yours. We love our moms and are grateful for their roles in our lives, but there is absolutely no reason why we must be tethered to their paradigm of mother-hood. Our path to motherhood was likely different, so we must give ourselves grace and create an experience that reflects our uniqueness. Chances are that if you struggle to receive, at some level, your mom does/did, too. You can honor your uniqueness as a woman and mother while, at the same time, setting a new example for what it means to receive for the women in your family who will come after you. *Yes, this is the transformative power of receiving.*

ROSANNE, WHAT DOES RECEIVING ACTUALLY LOOK LIKE?

Now let's explore what receiving during this pregnancy can look like. For me as a teacher and mentor, it centers on self-care at a fundamental level. It is beyond the occasional spa day here and there. It is about preparing your life and lifestyle for this baby by securing the consistent support you need in the home, the support you need from those around you, and an unrelenting commitment to putting Mommy's oxygen mask on first. The mistake most women make is they wait to address all of this until *after* their baby is born, largely for the reasons we discussed earlier—the *mirepoix of misery*, a.k.a. guilt, shame, and fear. You are pregnant; now is the perfect time to begin marshaling the resources you will need to enjoy this experience. And, just in case you need a reminder, your life is about to change in a huge way. You will have to get better at allocating your time and resources so that you can be the mom you say you want to be.

Here are some examples of what receiving can look like:

- **Begin ordering your groceries from a delivery service.** Once you have a newborn, you and your partner are going to be too tired for last-minute jaunts to the grocery store.
- **Find a consistent and trustworthy housekeeper** who will make your house as clean and sparkly as you want it to be—have no shame in your OCD game! If you want your towels folded to Martha Stewart perfection, make no apologies!
- **Consider hiring a house manager.** This is someone who will come in and do your laundry, meal prep, tidying, watering plants, errand-running, decorating, gift-wrapping, and travel arrangement-making and will make sure your house runs smoothly so the wheels don't come flying off. This will end all the bickering about socks on the floor and whose turn it is to do chores. Eliminate that fight by having a house manager! Getting our own house manager was transformative for the Austin Family. Quality time together is priceless. Delegate so you can celebrate in peace with the newest member of your family!
- **Schedule weekly two-hour Mommy Mental Breaks.** I know this may seem impossible, but it is essential. Having time to recharge your batteries and do something just for you—like stare at the wall or even window-shop—will refresh your energy so you have more to give to your precious baby (without burnout).
- **When friends and relatives ask how they can help, don't hold back.** Tell the people around you exactly

what you need. Stop judging yourself and silencing your needs. Those who truly want to help will be much happier to help you in a way that is meaningful rather than in whatever way *you* settle for.

- **Tell your partner what you need.** Now is not the time to beat around the bush. Your body is going through major changes, and while, indeed, you are your own special version of Superwoman, we all have our limits. While your partner can't participate in the physical experience of carrying this child, one of the ways you can include them is by letting them meet your needs—physical and emotional. Tell them what you want!

EXERCISING PREGNANT PRIVILEGE

What I have given you here is just a start and a lovely segue into the topic of "Pregnant Privilege." When you have been dreaming of being pregnant for any amount of time, unquestionably, one of the things that have crossed your mind is the special care and consideration that pregnant women *receive*. (Yes, there's that word again.) Throughout time, pregnant women have been shown reverence and deference and have been celebrated as "magical creatures," endowed with the ability to carry a precious life. Now that you are in that place, you—yes, you, Mama—get to partake in **Pregnant Privilege**.

I know that the word "privilege" may come with a bit of a tainted connotation, but I urge you to reject that notion. There's nothing negative about it. I see it as the celebration of a miracle. It doesn't make you better or worse than anyone—just different, and thereby warranting special care.

I know that the fiercely independent side of you may scoff at this, but let me remind you that the impulse to do everything on your own with no help or special consideration is your masculine energy. We all have masculine and feminine energy that moves through us. The masculine is the doer, while the feminine is the receiver. This has nothing to do with gender stereotypes. Rather, it is about the nature of our energy as human beings. You are pregnant. You are engaging in a natural process that is the most feminine thing you can possibly do, as only biological females get pregnant and have babies. Making babies is the essence of creative, feminine energy. Bask in this, Mama! Exercising Pregnant Privilege is about allowing yourself to be treated with extra special care, not because you are weak or incapable, but because life is precious and communities from the dawn of time have rallied around women to support them at this truly wonderful time. Let people open doors for you. Let people carry your groceries. Let the people around you celebrate this miracle by being there for you! Accept the complimentary upgrade from economy to first class when you fly.

This is also part of you taking excellent care of this child as your body changes and as your physical and emotional needs change. Take rests when you need to. Seriously, who is going to bag on the pregnant lady for taking a break or not feeling up to a girls' night out?

I know you might be shaking your head, saying, *That's nice for everyone else, Rosanne, but I can't because:*

- I don't have time.
- I don't have the money for the *schmancy* things you are talking about—I spent it "all" on having this baby.
- People will think I'm a diva.
- *Only I* am best suited to do the "home" stuff.
- It's too hard to train someone.
- I don't want a "strange" person in my house near my baby.
- People will think I can't hack it.
- If my mom did it, so can I.

- If I have someone else doing those things, I will miss out.

Chances are, you've got one or more of these stories running around and wreaking havoc on any excitement that you might be feeling at the prospect of exercising Pregnant Privilege. Don't worry. This is something that can be changed quickly, through the development of an Abundant Pregnancy Mindset.

ABUNDANT PREGNANCY MINDSET

I am sure that, through your reading and personal development during your fertility journey, you heard ethereal-sounding terms like *abundance* bantered about within the context of manifestation, law of attraction, and mindset. When it comes to the **Abundant Pregnancy Mindset** that I am talking about, we are really homing in on a heightened level of receptivity to receiving, which makes it a corollary concept to the Pregnant Privilege concept I shared earlier. It is essentially the belief that, because of your unique state of being pregnant, the Universe will naturally be sending you even more resources, support, and opportunities for growth than ever before. Put another way, it's like saying, "Of course there are increased blessings for me—I'm carrying a precious new life!" It's the leap from "Oh, you didn't have to do that," to an emphatic, "Why, yes, I will take a double scoop of that goodness—one for me and one for my baby!"

The Abundant Pregnancy Mindset is rooted in a foundation that there is more than enough good to go around for everyone —whether it is blessings, money, resources, love, time, or attention—*and* in the acknowledgment that pregnant women are deserving of extra attention and care due to the very important job they are doing. I see this mindset as one that honors the very real magic that is happening spiritually and physically for a woman who is pregnant and for those who get to be in her presence. Even now, five years after my pregnancy with my son Asher, I get uber-giddy around pregnant women because I see their undeniable glow, their energy of potential and possibility, and I remember how good that felt. Everything about pregnancy revolves around growth, expansion, and possibility. Let this reality help you push beyond your excuses and fear-based limitations about what you "can" or "can't" have during this precious time in your life. Exercise your Pregnant Privilege and open your heart and mind to receive as much as you desire with an Abundant Pregnancy Mindset.

RECEIVING HELPED ANNE-SOPHIE CARRY HER MIRACLE GIRL TO TERM

I know that all of this "receiving stuff" may be a lot to wrap your head around, and your mind may be shouting, "But Rosanne, what does this really look like? And can I really have that?!" This is why I am going to share a quick story about another one of my Miracle Mamas, Anne-Sophie. A French technology executive, Anne-Sophie came to me after struggling with recurrent miscarriage. There was nothing she wanted more than to be a mom, but she found herself feeling trapped in a demanding corporate job that was running her down. She longed for more freedom and for a chance to focus on healing her body and mind so she could call in the miracle she knew was meant for her.

Part of our work together was crushing the belief that she couldn't "have it all"—meaning have a flexible career, excellent pay, romance, travel, and life on her terms. Once she started challenging her old beliefs and applying what I was teaching her, something incredible happened: she got pregnant naturally *and* was offered the exact job she desired, which gave her the autonomy, flexibility, and sexy title she craved. She received both at virtually the same time!

She agonized over whether it was all "too much," and she began to worry that something would go wrong because of all the blessings that were coming into her life. This is where having her practice Pregnant Privilege, supported by her Abundant Pregnancy Mindset, was critical. She gave herself more grace, took the time off that she needed, got the help around the house that she wanted, and moved through her full-term pregnancy with ease.

Anne-Sophie's courage to allow herself to receive empowered her to not only feel more supported than ever, but to develop trust in a good and abundant Universe, as well as reigniting her trust in herself, her body, and the daughter she knew was meant for her. In fact, just moments ago, as I was writing these words, Anne-Sophie texted me a picture of her gummy-smiled three-month-old baby girl. Can you see why opening your heart to receiving is so incredibly important?

REVEL IN RIDICULOUS RECEIVING

Now that I have given you some powerful insight into receiving and why it is critically important to your well-being, as well as examples of how it might look in your life, let's shift our attention to making it your reality. This is where I will share an exercise that I often give to my Miracle Mamas: **Reveling in Ridiculous Receiving.** The process is simple, so don't overcomplicate it:

- Grab a piece of paper or flip to a page in your journal and draw two lines from top to bottom, creating three columns.
- At the top of each column, write (one word per column) the following words: *Receive, Excuse, Date of Completion.*

- In the *Receive* column, write at least ten things that you would *love* to receive. Trust your heart here and drop any judgments. What would excite you like crazy to receive during your pregnancy? Go crazy. Have fun. Maybe a Hawaiian babymoon? A super sexy bougie stroller? A designer diaper bag? A reality TV–worthy baby shower? Refuse to pump the brakes. Be generous.

- In the *Excuse* column, write the #1 excuse you will use to *not* have this thing. Notice how it feels in your body to write out each excuse. Do you feel your spirit suffocate? Do you hear the voice of a parent who lives by lack and scarcity? Do you hear the voice of a judgy friend who loves to be a martyr? Make a decision that, to honor the abundant and kind Universe that brought you this miracle pregnancy, you will silence your excuses and *receive*.

- In the *Date* column, write down the exact date by which you will get/do the thing or have the experience you desire to receive.

- Finally, allow yourself to receive each of the items on your list in the *Receive* column. But don't receive sheepishly. Allow yourself to *revel* in the joy, excitement, and beauty of what you are receiving. Let your soul delight in treating yourself and this baby. Give yourself permission to receive so much that it feels almost ridiculous. By doing so, you will gain tangible evidence that not only does receiving feel like warm sunshine on your face, but you can receive and live to tell the tale.

It is my sincere prayer that you now understand why receiving is the secret to pregnancy bliss. This has nothing to do with being "high maintenance" or incapable. It's about a righteous celebration of a miracle and allowing yourself to take up more space in this life—and you are going to need it because not only are you growing, but your family is as well. Spiritual, emotional, and physical starvation will leave you without the fuel you need for the next phase in your life. Receive, Mama, receive.

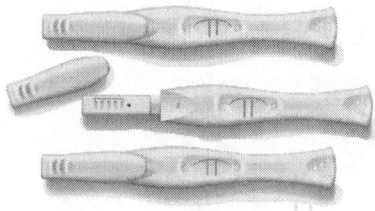

Chapter 6

Bump Squad, Pregnancy Style

There's a funny thing that can happen on the way to Mama Town: the relationships with the people around you can get, shall we say, *interesting*. With eight years of coaching under my belt, I've observed that women generally fall into one of two categories when it comes to how we've managed our relationships while trying to conceive. We've either treated trying to conceive like a deep, dark secret, so we go about our business like Bruce Wayne and Batman, hiding the truth about what we are going through from even those closest to us, or we've worn our hearts on our sleeves to the point where (at least in our minds), people know us as *the sad girl who can't get pregnant*. While certainly there are myriad combinations and shades of each of these generalizations, chances are you will identify quickly with one end of the spectrum or another. Thus, we are presented with the interesting question of how to transition out of those shame-laden labels into an entirely new identity as *the pregnant lady*. This and its tentacles of related complexities are what we will be exploring in this chapter.

YOUR PREGNANCY BUMP SQUAD

Let me start by briefly explaining the term *Bump Squad*. What I refer to as your Bump Squad is a core group of people who you have come to trust and rely on during your fertility journey. In my first book, this referred to those who you counted on for support—both emotional and physical—as well as for treatments and care while you were trying to conceive. Some of these relationships were personal ones, others professional. A Bump Squad is meant to be an evolving group of people who love you without question and believe in you unconditionally.

The question when it comes to selecting your Bump Squad is simple: *Does this person believe in me?* I chose the words *believe in* carefully because it's about respect for your vision and discernment as both a human being and a mother-to-be. When someone *believes in* you, there is no need (on their part) to try to control you or push their beliefs on you. Someone who believes in you honors your right to have your own experience and will lovingly weigh in if you ask them to. There's an air of inherent or earned trust that eliminates any confusion about who is in the driver's seat and any need to battle over who is "right." Those on your Bump Squad see you as an equal, not as someone who needs to be saved or pitied. It is a distinct honor to invite someone onto your Bump Squad, and those who are invited should be aware of the hallowed land upon which they tread. They essentially get a front row seat to watching a woman make her dreams come true. *It's the best show in town!*

Now that you know what a Bump Squad is, I want to zero in

on an important aspect of it. Your Bump Squad is intended to be a group of people around you that evolves. People will come and go. When they do, it's not because you are necessarily angry or displeased with them. Instead, it's about allowing your Bump Squad to reflect where you are on this journey. You may also find that it's important to enforce different boundaries with different people at different times. I called this **The Velvet Rope Technique** in my first book—yep, like the velvet rope that you might see outside of a nightclub or movie premiere. The Velvet Rope Technique is about making gentle (but clear) adjustments to who is granted admittance to your inner circle of support at any given time. *(That's why I describe this technique as a velvet rope, not barbed wire!)* Some may be moved in and out of your Bump Squad rather fluidly, while others may be moved outside the velvet rope entirely... and stay there. None of this is about judging someone's value as a human being. It is about making your well-being, on all levels, a priority. You may find that now that you're pregnant, those who were part of your Bump Squad while you were trying to conceive no longer play as big of a role (if any). If you find yourself in a place where people's roles are changing in your life, that's perfectly okay, and it's to be expected.

Chances are that, as you read these words, you have a sense of who your Bump Squad is—and maybe even a sense of some "upgrades" you'd like to make. It's also important to note here that your Bump Squad could be a few people... or it may just be you! As with most things, it's more about the *quality* of the members than it is about the quantity. With that said, here's what pruning your Bump Squad may look like in concrete terms:

- Letting go of your super awesome but worst-case-scenario-oriented fertility doctor.
- Exiting fertility-related online groups, message boards, or in-person support groups. (This may feel

like disloyal, turncoat behavior at first, but it is likely one of the smartest things you can do to cement your transition into *mama-to-be*. Just remember that any judgment of your choices has more to do with the person judging than it does with you.)

- Excluding those who, for better or worse, love to share stories of woe and tragedy, punctuating them with the disclaimer of, *"But I'm sure it won't happen to you."* (You know the type—every family or friend group has one!) *Cut 'em off like a dead branch!*

- Reducing your exposure to family members or friends who are competitive and feed on comparison— particularly if they, too, are expecting! (Some think it's super cute to be pregnant at the same time as our friends and family… *but is it?*)

- Releasing those who, for some reason or another, it just feels natural to let go of!

The pruning process, generally speaking, happens in one of three ways. (1) There is a natural parting of ways where nothing but thanks is exchanged and you seamlessly go about your merry ways, (2) a new boundary is set in the wake of an irksome incident, or (3) there is a boiling point moment, lines are crossed, battleships are positioned, and each side makes definitive statements about "that" never happening again. This means that pruning can, in essence, involve gradations of, "Till next time," "I will be seeing less of you," or "Yeah, buh-bye." Whatever the case may be, remember that a natural aspect of pruning (as with trees) is new growth, for both you and the pruned. This is not a bad thing. It opens up space for new people to come into both of your lives.

You may be wondering, "How exactly does one go about pruning?" I am sure that question brings up some anxiety, as our imaginations can take us through a jaunt down Caustic

Conflict Lane, but don't fall for that nonsense. Pruning doesn't require dramatic showdowns. As I said earlier, it generally happens in one of the three ways I detailed, but what unifies those potentialities is *a conversation.* Yup, *you are going to have to talk to people.*

Most people shy away from uncomfortable situations without appreciating that such unfinished business or unresolved conflict only creates more stress. Mama doesn't need that —nor does she need overly complicated machinations. If you are parting ways on super great terms because it makes sense to and it's time, thank the person and let them know that you will reach out again should the need arise. Have a friend or family member who is otherwise awesome and just happened to "step in it"? Just say, "I know you probably didn't mean this, but when you did _____, it didn't feel great to me. Will you please keep that in mind?" Or maybe an opinionated aunt decides she wants to bring up choices from your past and says, "Gee, well, you did put your career before your family, so let's hope your baby doesn't have any problems." You can simply respond with, "Hey, Aunt_____, thanks for your concern. I am super proud of my choices in this life, and my baby is perfect. When you are ready to share in that vision, you can join the rest of us in celebrating this blessing." Say that preceding statement like a Mama Bear drawing a boundary, not a judge handing down a sentence. People don't know what they don't know! This journey has impacted you in ways others may never understand. Your values and insights may begin to look very different from those of the people around you. That's not a judgment; it's a reality. Keep your pruning conversations simple, direct, and focused on being a celebration of self-determination. Can you see why pruning is so important?

REFINING YOUR BUMP SQUAD FOR PREGNANCY

Whatever the state of your current Bump Squad, you will have quite an opportunity to revisit the subject of who is on it and the role they will play now that you are pregnant. While this is an intensely exciting time full of change, it also presents some rather hairy issues that you must navigate with those closest to you.

It all begins seconds after you see the two lines, while the wave of shrieking joy washes over you—*OMG, who am I going to tell?!* It doesn't matter how many times you rehearsed this moment in your head and what you thought you would do; most of that goes out the window as you hoot, howl, and holler about finally being "here." Of course, you will tell your partner immediately, but what about everyone else?

Here is where the Shakespearean drama in our heads begins. *To tell or not to tell? Who makes the cut… and when?* For some in your life, the answer is obvious, but for others, not so much. There are also layers of complexity we create for ourselves as we try to gauge nuances like timing and even merit! Sometimes we can even feel like we "owe" certain people access to this information simply based on who they are and societal or cultural expectations.

You Are in Charge of Your Pregnancy

What I encourage you to do if you find yourself wrestling with how much to share and with whom you choose to share it is to take a moment to acknowledge that you are in an entirely new time in your life. There will be new rules and boundaries to consider for everyone. The terrain on this journey unquestionably changes as you get closer to the promised land. You may find that people in your life become strangely possessive and covetous when it comes to the details about your success and what happens now that you are pregnant. As your baby's Mama Bear, you've got to stay focused on who is in charge: *you.*

The whole truth is that you don't owe anyone anything on this journey. You are under no obligation to share details that you don't care to, and you are 100% in control of the timing and manner in which anyone finds out about your pregnancy. Sadly, many love to take this information and put it on blast as a means of making themselves feel significant. It's quite entitled behavior that you have no need to support. I see this a lot when it comes to relations with in-laws. If no one has said this to you, let me be clear: the information about your pregnancy, how you got "here," and what lies ahead belongs to you. Yes, your partner (if you are partnered) may want to share it with their family, but you want to have a baseline understanding that your privacy and your wishes about the dissemination of this information must be respected. Conflict can be avoided when we establish clear and firm boundaries up front—and setting them early will pay off because there will be many challenges to those boundaries as your pregnancy progresses.

Letting Go of Old Labels

This leads us to a much-needed discussion about letting go of the labels you may have been emblazoned with in the past. During your fertility journey, I'm willing to bet that you picked up some labels along the way like "geriatric," "recurrent loss," "hard case," "high risk," "complicated," or "needy." Whether they realize it or not, the people who helped us get "here" often hold on to those notions long after you've let them go. These labels shape their opinions, motivate their behaviors, and can cause them to approach your pregnancy with fear and anxiety that maybe *you* don't even have!

Whatever the case may be, it's important to begin to shape a new narrative and make sure that your growing bump is surrounded by the right squad. When it comes to releasing the labels of the past, I have found that taking a direct and decisive approach—with *all* the members of your Squad—is best. No pomp or circumstance is needed. Simply let them know that, while certain labels may have been applied to you in the past, you simply choose not to live by them any longer. You are pregnant! The statistics are no longer relevant. You beat the odds and are therefore an "outlier," in the best possible way. Tell them in a clear and concise way that you choose to focus on this victory—not on the labels of the past. You've moved into a new phase, and if they want to stay on your Bump Squad, they will need to as well. *You aren't "that" girl anymore!*

Does this mean that you are denying your past? No. Does this mean that you don't take some elements from your history to inform your approach to this pregnancy? No. You are simply making the conscious decision to shed past labels that no longer apply to your glorious current reality. Again, this isn't denial— this is a conscious choice about where you focus your energy *and* that you are not going to live in the past.

What I've just shared applies to your Bump Squad—but what about *you*? In case there's still a niggling part of you that wants to cling to those labels, despite the work we've done together in the previous chapters, let me help you quickly and decisively decapitate that dragon now. Tormenting yourself with those labels inherently takes you out of the present and drags your butt back to the past. Your baby is not in the past. Your baby is here with you now, in the present, as you read these pages. You get to choose here and now who you are going to be. Are you going to spend the forty weeks of your pregnancy as "the girl who can't get and stay pregnant," or are you going to be "the woman who beat the odds"? The choice is yours—but you can probably feel the dramatic difference between the two states of mind as you read those words. One anchors you to the past. The other is a forward-focused celebration of where you are headed. There is truth in the adage "Where your attention goes, energy flows." To whom are you going to give your precious energy—to this baby, or to your fears from the past? Choose wisely.

You've fought long and hard to get here. Drop those old labels like a hot potato and rock your new one as *the glorious pregnant lady*. Now, if that little talking-to doesn't whip you into shape, review the work we did in the previous chapters—no shame, Mama. This takes a little practice, but it will get easier.

Getting the Side-Eye about Your Success?

Another aspect of navigating relationships with the people in your life as you move through your pregnancy—whether those people are specifically on your Bump Squad or not—is dealing with the suspicions and judgments that those around you might have about the very existence of this pregnancy. While it may be hard to fathom that anyone would harbor any disdain for someone making their dreams a reality, there are likely some people in your life who may be giving you the side-eye. Whether you just *suspect* this is happening or have painful confirmation of it, rest assured that you are not alone. When you pull away from the pack and refuse to live your life in an unfulfilled and mediocre way, there will be those who hate on you, no matter how heartwarming your story is. There are inevitably going to be those in your life for whom your success only amplifies their level of regret over the dreams they abandoned. As a result, they may lash out in various ways—some subtle, others blatant. I see this happen most often in the following ways:

- Sneering, judgy comments about fertility treatments being "unnatural" or "unholy"

- Weird, glaringly illogical comparisons to other members of the family or circle of friends who didn't have to "resort" to having fertility support
- Shaming or "I could never do that"s around your specific choices
- Whispers about your child being "different" than the others—particularly if you chose to use a donor egg or sperm
- Passive aggressive comments like "Wow, I couldn't imagine having kids at your age…"
- Lack and scarcity-laden quips like "It must be nice to spend that kind of money on having a kid. I hope you set some aside to raise them!"

There are a zillion other variations of these statements, but they all have one thing in common: you are somehow "wrong" for going about your journey in the way that you did. It doesn't matter what you did or how you did it, the haters in your life will always find a way to make a dig. Even if you are blessed enough to not have haters in your life, chances are, your Saboteurs will make good use of similar fodder to try to make you wrong for your choices. When they do (and they are sneaky!) just go back to chapter 3 and review the Woman, You Did Good Letter you wrote to yourself for being the woman who went the distance.

I'm the Only One Pregnant… I'm "Late" to the Game

Another interesting situation you may face during your pregnancy is potentially being the only one in your friend group or peer group who is pregnant. If you are anything like me, most of your friends already had their kids or had made the decision not to have them. When I got pregnant, I felt strangely like the odd one out—not judged, necessarily, but perhaps "late to the game." While most of the weirdness I felt was completely of my own creation, I do distinctly recall getting some funny looks that seemed to find the novelty of my pregnancy, on the eve of my mid-forties, condescendingly charming. It was as if they were saying, "Oh, how cute, she's one of those!" I was clearly out of sync with the normal flow of how life is "supposed" to go. While others were waxing rhapsodical about their kids leaving the house, my husband and I were decorating our nursery!

If you find yourself in a similar place, there's one thing you must keep in mind: you don't do life like everyone else. I'm willing to bet one of my beloved vintage Chanel bags that having your baby isn't the only way you've bucked tradition. You've always been "different," in the best possible way, and you know it. Embrace being an anomaly—whether it is having a baby "later," or in a way that is different from those in your life. Your timing is perfect, and your way is divine!

Bottom Line? You Are Mama Bear

I've been alluding to this "Mama Bear" thing throughout this book, but now we are going to explore what that actually means and how it can empower you. There's a pivotal fact that you can choose to embrace—and I unabashedly encourage you to. *You are Mama Bear.* That means that it doesn't matter one lick what anyone else thinks about you, how you got here, or where you are headed in this pregnancy. You are this child's mother, and that makes you the sole authority.

This statement of fact isn't to diminish the role of fathers and partners; they play a vital role indeed. However, it is a statement that honors biological and spiritual truth. You are the vessel through which this child passes into the material world. Your body is growing a miracle. Everything you do impacts this child—including the food you eat, the care you get, and the company you keep. You know what's right for you, and you know what's right for this child. Bottom line? This means you are the sole arbiter of what does and does not happen. Your way gets to be the highway! From what you want to do for your baby shower (if you choose to have one) to the special dietary requests you desire to have honored, you get to do "this" your way.

Some may see this level of resolve as your irretrievable descent into a narcissistic abyss, but it's not. You are Mama Bear, and the proverbial buck stops with you. I know you have probably been conditioned to see this kind of resolve as selfishly one-sided, and even if there's part of you jumping for joy at reading these words, you may experience momentary pangs of guilt. All of that is perfectly fine, but stay focused. This is your dream, and *you* did the work to get here. You would be well within your rights to consider other people's opinions, but in the end, Mama Bear has the final say. None of that is selfish or wrong. It is you establishing your boundaries and stating your wishes as your baby's mama. Question the motives of anyone who tries to suggest otherwise!

You may as well get used to taking the lead when it comes to caring for your child—they will be here sooner than you think. Start practicing Mama Bear-ness now!

THE PROS ON YOUR BUMP SQUAD

Up to this point, we have talked mostly about the personal relationships included in your Bump Squad. Now it's time to turn our attention to the professionals you select to be by your side during your pregnancy.

Mama, you want to select professionals who will truly support you and look beyond your possibly "shady" fertility past (I say that with love.). The last thing you need is someone who will constantly be fearmongering based on your past. For sure you will want to get the best possible care that will take your needs into account, but that's not the same as having your past cast a shadow on your present. You want professionals who will give you the facts, help you with solutions, and cheer you on the whole way. Trust me, you don't want Chicken Little with you at every appointment and scan or, even worse, in the delivery room! Find an OB/GYN and other professionals who love fertility success stories and acknowledge that women of all ages go on to have healthy, happy pregnancies. Bedside manner matters. Trust your instincts and find those with whom you resonate.

PRUNING HELPED DR. NINA GET AND STAY PREGNANT

To put what I've shared here in very real terms, I want to share the story of one of my most beloved ladies, Dr. Nina. A medical doctor with a highly sought-after specialty, Dr. Nina was used to having her voice heard and respected. When it came to her family of origin, however, she might as well have been a high school dropout living on her parents' couch. Nothing was ever enough for her parents. It didn't matter how many lives she saved or how many fellowships and papers she had published; she was always going to be the odd one out.

She had been a bit of a rebel since she was little. Her family was frightened by and judgmental of her "black sheep" ways, and this extended well into her adulthood, particularly when she found her partner. Not only was he outside of her culture, but their committed relationship was not a marriage. This sent shudders of shame down her parents' collective spine, and they made their disapproval well-known to Nina. On top of the disapproval of her parents, Nina found herself being chided by her colleagues for trying to have a baby "at her age" and with her diminished ovarian reserve. At first, Dr. Nina was hurt by this lack of support from those closest to her, but I coached her to remember that she was going to be a mom and might as well start acting like a Mama Bear in anticipation of having her baby. She began tapping into her power as a Mama Bear-to-be and quickly started to assert new boundaries with family and colleagues—letting both know that her personal choices were not subject to debate. It wasn't easy, but with practice, Dr. Nina developed her confidence and stopped letting herself be bullied by unsolicited commentary from family and colleagues.

Despite the overwhelming disapproval all around, Dr. Nina and her partner decided to trust themselves and their hearts to have their baby. In the face of insanely negative statistics, Dr. Nina got pregnant naturally and carried her precious son to term. Her family never quite came around, but, based on the serene smile she had on her face in the delivery room (she texted me a pic), what they thought didn't end up mattering much—*she now had a family of her own*. She was so glad she held her ground and allowed herself to trust her Mama Bear energy, just like I had taught her. My prayer for you is that you will do the same.

BE MAMA BEAR NOW

To help you find and assert your Mama Bear energy, I want to share an exercise with you here, one that I call **Summon Mama Bear Energy**. Here's how it works:

- Take out a clean sheet of paper or open to a new page in your journal, and grab something to write with.
- Draw a line down the center of the page.
- At the top of the first column, write *Their Expectations*. At the top of the second column, write *What Mama Bear Wants*.
- Under the *Their Expectations* column, make a list of expectations that others have of you right now. That

could be expectations from your employer, friends, family, partner, or even your treatment team. What are the expressed and implied expectations that they have of you? Has someone assumed *they* will plan your baby shower—without considering what you want? Does your physician expect you to induce labor early, just because you are "older"? Does your partner insist upon naming your child after their father, even though you *hate* that name? Does your employer expect you to work at the same level you did prior to your pregnancy, without considering possible risks? Write down all "their expectations."

- Under the *What Mama Bear Wants* column, next to the corresponding *Their Expectations*, write what you desire in that situation. Don't consider *how* you will make your desire manifest—just write what you want, without any editing or judgment. As you write what you want, just know that your Saboteurs will come at you hard. These limiting beliefs will try to make you feel bad for writing your desires down. Reject those notions. Remember, you are Mama Bear!

- Read the information in both columns again. Circle the items that are most important to you. What are you most committed to? It's important to know where you will draw hard lines. There may be some topics where the gap between what people expect and what you want is not that wide. You may desire to take a more flexible stance there if it feels good to you. Either way, use this exercise to **"Exorcise" the Expectations** that are out of alignment with what you truly value. When I say "exorcise an expectation," I mean reject it. Boot it out of your life. Make it clear to the holder of that expectation that it's a no-go for you. While you may love that person, you don't love the

expectation, and you refuse to accept it. Worried
about this being confrontational or awkward?
Summon your Mama Bear Energy, just like I
taught you.

Navigating the other people in your life during your pregnancy isn't always going to be easy, but it is a chance for you to
rediscover and assert your personal sovereignty as a woman and
a mother-to-be. Let your intuition guide you here, and be
patient with yourself. You may find that there will be those who
opt out of this stage in your journey, and that's perfectly okay.
Take a moment to thank them for the role they played and keep
your heart open to the possibility of them coming back into your
life at another time. We are ever-evolving beings! Take comfort
in having people around you during your pregnancy who believe
in you, toss out the old labels, make space for your growth, and
genuinely love to see you thrive.

Here's to your new Bump Squad, pregnancy style!

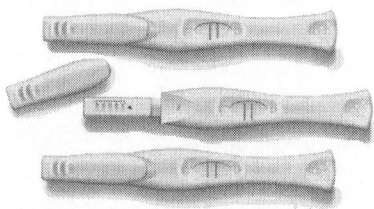

Chapter 7

Babe, There's Three of Us in This Relationship

There is a distinct moment, after all the initial excitement and fanfare of finding out you are pregnant, mellows out when you and your partner realize that it isn't just the two of you in this family anymore. There is a little human being who is in the process of making their way to you... *and they will be moving in very soon!* This presents couples with real and distinct challenges that I believe fall into three categories: physical, emotional, and the value-based practical.

Be careful here to not immediately read and interpret the word *challenges* as negative. Nothing we are discussing here is negative in and of itself, *unless of course it goes unprepared for,* which is why I am doing you a massive solid right now by dragging it out of the shadows.

THE PHYSICAL

Where the Drift Begins

You've got a lot going on in your body right now, Mama. Your partner doesn't. This might be so obvious that it gets overlooked. We aren't going to make that mistake here. The reality is that you are carrying this pregnancy and, for the next forty weeks, there will be demands made on your body that are unrelenting. You don't get a break from pregnancy-related sickness or fatigue, your body is changing at a rapid pace, and everything you do impacts this little one you are carrying in one way or another. For your partner, on the other hand, physically, it's business as usual. Your pregnancy is a concrete reality for you—you feel it. But for your husband or partner, they hear the words "pregnant" and "baby," and they understand them intellectually, but the emotional and physical reality haven't quite caught up yet—and probably won't for a while... until, of course, your bump becomes unmistakable.

If you find yourself in that place, rest assured it's completely normal. Your baby is growing inside of y-o-u. Therefore, you are acutely aware of how quickly things are changing and how really real they are. I know you understand this, but it bears reinforcement. Sometimes couples get so caught up in the initial excitement that this reality gets overlooked. Then, down the road, tension builds, and you and your partner may find yourselves wondering if you are going to be able to "hack" this pregnancy and parenting "thing." I know that may sound dramatic at first, but mark my words, the thought will cross your mind—particularly as you begin to see the disparity between the relative freedom your partner has and the relative lack you're feeling, as the demands on your body are greater and the restrictions on your lifestyle and activities begin to increase. I know you are super glad to have this "problem" and be in this position, but trust me, you will have momentary breaks from that bliss.

Important side note: It's fascinating to me how people think that the moment you are pregnant, a bump appears. They don't realize that you might make it through your first trimester of pregnancy without any visible protrusion from your abdomen! Why does this matter in the context of possible challenges in your relationship? For all intents and purposes, to your partner, *you look the same!* They don't see you doing the pregnant lady waddle (yet), you are probably keeping up with your daily life and work, and you are more than likely still wearing your regular clothes. People forget that even in the absence of a visible bump, your hormones are raging, you are dealing with some unpleasant pregnancy symptoms to varying degrees, and, as delighted as you are to be pregnant, your body is changing at such a breakneck pace that sometimes you don't know up from down.

This lack of immediate physical indicators that you are pregnant can cause your partner, *as crazy as it sounds*, to treat you exactly as they did before, with no special consideration for your pregnancy. In the fog of the first trimester crazy, this can unfairly cast a shadow of inconsiderate selfishness on your partner. More than a few of my ladies have run into this issue and found themselves growing angry with their partners for suggesting that they engage in their usual responsibilities or activities when they are in no practical condition to do those things. Seriously, you might look "fine" but feel like you ran two marathons with a bag of bricks on your chest! You also might not be so down with going on a weekend of wine tasting with friends when not only are you avoiding alcohol, but the smell of wine makes you want to hurl.

If some of this is bubbling up for you, Mama, don't just write your partner off as utterly tone-deaf. They simply need to be reminded of your *pregnant reality*—and often. This is where honest communication is critical. You are no less of a badass just because you are asking for some slack while your body adjusts to each new stage of your pregnancy. Nor are you making excuses when you just want to sleep! Take responsibility for lovingly educating your partner about where you are physically so that, while indeed the two of you are having two very different physical experiences right now, those differences don't cause a drift or a rift.

What Is Happening to My Woman?!

When it comes to the physical changes/challenges that you are experiencing as your pregnancy progresses, there is a real possibility that they are downright scary to your partner. Your partner might not have ever seen you mowed down (even temporarily) by fatigue or illness. It's also possible that, as your body changes, which may include weight gain or less mobility (as often happens later in pregnancy) or you develop special needs (such as bed rest, gestational diabetes, or other pregnancy-related conditions, and possibly being designated as "high risk"), your partner can feel helpless and hamstrung. I have even come across instances when a partner develops anxiety regarding birth and delivery, along with the inherent risk of unforeseen complications. While of course these things are happening *to you*, it's not ridiculous to consider that they are unsettling or frightening to your partner—who loves you very much and, I would dare say, would be devastated if something happened to you.

While your partner is extremely excited about this baby, this may be the first time they ever considered your mortality or their own. Pregnancy is a huge leap into "adulting," regardless of how mature your partner may seem.

If your partner seems more tense than usual or begins treating you like you are made of glass, be sure to check in with them and see if this might be happening for them so you can address it together, rather than letting it create a wedge between you.

When Sexy Says Goodbye

Couples who have struggled to conceive may find that, once their baby makes their presence known, what was once a very active playground may turn into a postapocalyptic ghost town. Plain and simple? I've seen Miracle Mamas become downright terrified of having sex. They fear the act will somehow dislodge their baby and they will face the heartbreak of a loss, after having just made it to Mama Town. Much to her partner's dismay, Mama may forgo a roll in the hay in order to keep the Golden Ticket of her pregnancy squarely in her protective hands.

I'm not here to say this is somehow irrational or unwarranted. Every woman's situation and pregnancy history is different and must be valued, but there is no question that taking a position such as this presents the physical intimacy of your relationship with some very real challenges. This is not to say that this fear is one-sided, either! You may find that your male partner has his own level of terror around the subject and may suddenly decline your advances.

Whatever the case may be, when it comes to the physical changes you are experiencing and any anxiety you and/or your partner have about sex and intercourse, woman, you've got to summon your Mama Bear energy and have a conversation. Calling in Mama Bear energy here is not about mothering your partner or condescending to them (I will say more about that in a bit). It's about taking responsibility for and showing some leadership in your relationship.

Some may be irritated by the thought of having to take on this role on top of "everything else," but it is critically important to do so *because your partner doesn't know what you are going through.*

Showing leadership isn't synonymous with emasculation. It's demonstrating some emotional maturity and ownership over the trajectory of your relationship. Your partner may have no idea where to begin—*so help them!* Yes, it may feel like so much of this falls on your shoulders (and it does), but when you have open lines of communication with your partner, if you tell them where you stand and what you need from a place of love, compassion, and an orientation toward solutions, that burden has a better chance of becoming more evenly distributed. Don't overcomplicate this; just tell them precisely and concisely what your concerns are and how you'd like to approach the subject moving forward.

This could sound a lot like:

Hey, babe. I love you so much, and I'm so excited about this pregnancy. I have to admit that, with our struggles to conceive, I'm a little nervous about sex. This is not a rejection of you. I'm just a little scared. I would feel so much more at ease if we consulted our doctor first and then resumed our "regularly scheduled programming." Deal?

No blaming. No shaming. No withholding. Just truth. I find that, when navigating these sometimes-dicey waters with our partners, simplicity and honesty are best. Your fears about sexy time are going to come out one way or another, so you may as well spill the beans with love and an eye for improving communication and deepening your bond based on trust. Give your partner the benefit of the doubt. As I mentioned earlier, they may be even more cautious than you—give them a chance to be heard. You may just fall in love with them all over again. (Now, that's one heck of a come up!)

Keeping Your Partner Engaged… When It's All Happening to You

Continuing in our discussion about the physical changes in

your body and how your pregnancy can impact your relation-ship, there's also the challenge of keeping your partner excited and engaged when everything is "happening" to you. It can be hard for your partner to feel like they are an active participant when you are carrying the baby and everyone's attention, professional or otherwise, is pretty much on *you*. While this nuance can straddle both the physical and emotional, I catego-rize it more closely as a physical struggle because the solution lies in the actions that both of you take.

In the end, this is an invitation for your partner to take a more active and physical role than one might typically think. I hope that grabs your attention, because it's quite awesome. It's awesome because it requires you to do something we talked about in chapter 5. I know receiving is an area that my lovably hard-working, achievement-oriented ladies struggle with, but this is your chance to take it to the next level, Mama. When your baby comes, you will be so glad you did.

Giving your partner a more active and physical role in your pregnancy can look like the following:

- **Ask them to show up to every prenatal or follow-up appointment.** I'm serious about this. Ask them to show up whether it is "convenient" or not—and regardless of how long the appointment will be. I see a lot of women wave off this level of involvement initially, then later grow to resent their partner's absence. Don't do that! If you want them excited and engaged, then give them the chance to be excited and engaged. Every appointment will reveal more about this little person the two of you will be welcoming. This level of inclusion will deepen your partner's connection to what's really happening, and it lets them know you value their presence and support.

- **Let your partner *do* for you.** I realize this harkens back to chapter 5 again, and there's a reason for that: allowing your partner to *do* for you gives them a chance to contribute. The more they contribute, the more engaged they feel. Your partner will also learn, through *doing for you*, to begin to anticipate your needs, which is kind of the Holy Grail in relationships. If there is something you would normally do yourself, ask your partner to do it! Let them know how much it means to you! Ask them to get you ice cream. Let them go out of their way for one of your "pregnant lady" demands. Some partners will find it a badge of honor to go out of their way for you. Let them feel needed and wanted. Don't miss this chance, Mama. Remember, none of this makes you weak or needy.

- **Ask your partner to arrange for any prenatal or birthing classes.** I know your partner may balk at this at first, but giving them such an important job lets them know that you trust them. This also encourages your partner to do some prework and investigation into what considerations are right for your family. I know this is something you may have some strong opinions about, and you might think your partner is the *last* person who should be making these arrangements, but getting true engagement comes from your partner having some skin in the game, so let them at least bring you some options for these preparatory classes and receive those options with love and grace. Indeed, the decision on which classes are right for you is most likely a team effort, but let your partner bring you options!

- **Put your partner in charge of preparing the nursery.** This suggestion may initially make you shudder, but hear me out. I'm not saying that your partner must *design* the nursery—I'm sure you have some clear ideas about that—but let them execute on it. Think about any other important time in your life —people *love* to help and *love* to know they are doing something that has an impact. Chances are your partner would love to see the look on your face when they see they've helped you bring your nursery dreams to fruition.

- **Share your pregnancy highlight reel—*daily*.** Set aside one minute each day to let your partner know what's new and exciting in your pregnancy. I know this may sound weird at first, but rather than assuming what you share will be boring, repetitive, or "nothing new," just take a moment to share something about your pregnancy. Maybe you can't fit into your old jeans anymore, you finally see a little bump forming, or you can laugh about having a crying jag for no apparent reason! Let this be lighthearted. Engage your partner's curiosity. And, most importantly, don't let this turn into complaining. It's just you sharing a "day in the life" of sorts. Don't just assume they aren't interested. Some partners really look forward to these daily updates! Don't wait until things are super stressful before you include your partner. Make keeping them abreast of the situation part of your daily routine.

Love, these are just some ideas. There are so many ways that you can get your partner involved, but the most important are the ways that make you *both* feel seen and heard. Let your partner hear what you need and see that you are grateful!

THE EMOTIONAL

The other, perhaps thornier, area where I see couples drift and struggle during pregnancy is in how they interact emotionally. As your "we" becomes three (or more), the two of you are going to be making some rather significant emotional adjustments. You may have been used to your "couple" being a certain way, having certain routines, and engaging in certain dynamics that make things between you predictable and secure. While those won't totally go out the window, there will be some adjustment and unquestionably some anxiety about how the two of you will find your way through the most important "job" you will ever have. What I am sharing here are some of the most common places where I see couples needing to give each other some latitude and thoughtful attention.

Remember, getting in front of these issues is key, so if you read something here that feels quite pertinent, take the bull by the horns, Mama, and tell your partner how you feel. Invite them to do the same!

Your Hormones: Welcome to a Wild Ride

Let's face it: with the changes in your hormones, the reality of having made your pregnancy dreams come true, and the impact of any lingering fears and doubts, this is unquestionably an emotional time. It can be a bit confusing to feel excited, vulnerable, scared, and grateful all at the same time. If you find yourself in that place, join the club. Becoming a mom is as much an emotional process as it is a physical one. We have to reevaluate how we see ourselves, our partners, and our relationship to our work, as well as how we interact with others, among a zillion other considerations. Be patient with yourself. Be honest with your partner. If you are feeling a bit tender, let them know. If you need space, let them know. If you are scared out of your mind, let them know. Don't expect your partner to *fix it;* just ask them to witness it. If you want their help, other than just listening, then be sure to tell them that supporting you in that moment includes helping you find a solution. You may be very encouraged by what they come up with!

You may also find that during this time you find your unique "Mommy Mode." This is awesome, but a word of caution: be careful not to "mother" your partner. I raise this topic because I see women do this all the time. It reminds me of the old saying that "when you are a hammer, everything looks like a nail." Miracle Mamas can unwittingly engage in this dangerous behavior. They are pregnant, so everything looks like something that needs to be babied. *Not so when it comes to your partner!* Now is the time to let your partner rise to the occasion.

One of the biggest complaints I hear from women is that they feel like their partners have the "easy" part. The truth is, an uneven distribution of "work" in a relationship, particularly at this critical time, is a choice. Yes, it's a choice. While up to this point the two of you may have had the pattern of you taking on "everything," the time to break that nasty habit is now. Why? Because when you infantilize your partner, you block yourself from receiving the support you desire and block your partner from becoming the parent they desire to be. How can your partner step into their role as an equal co-parent when you treat them like a child or make things "easy" on them? They are an adult! There will come a time when you must step away and they will be taking care of the baby, so you may as well get used to trusting their judgment. Or prepare yourself for their disengagement and glaring looks of frustration. No one, not even children, enjoys being treated like a child!

Let your partner know what you need and expect them to meet those needs, or at least learn how to do so. Effective parenting with your partner requires a deep level of trust and communication, so let them grow into that role now.

Can you see now why we spent an entire chapter on receiving and how much of keeping your partner excited and engaged is about you taking a step back so *they* can do?

When Doubts about Your Relationship Creep In… Eeek!

This is also a time when many Miracle Mamas may begin to have some doubts about their relationships. I know you might not even want to think about this, but if you are honest, when you have been disappointed by your partner or they have not shown up the way you wanted them to, there was a sliver of this reality that poked through—and, chances are, it wasn't the first time. Here's what you must understand: when you are pregnant, the areas of your relationship that need attention only become amplified. While you might think your relationship is rom-com-worthy, there will be a time, perhaps a momentary slip-up, when it seems like someone abruptly switched the channel to a reality TV shouting match. It happens to the best of us!

Rather than taking this to mean that your relationship is doomed and you will end up being a miserable single parent, take the time now to speak plainly with your partner about roles and the division of labor. I don't care if you think you did this before you conceived. The time to do it again is *now*.

It might have been some time since you fantasized about what your roles would be and how things would "go." Now that the fantasy has become a reality, it's important to be sure you are both 100% on the same page. The simplest way to do that is just to have a conversation with your partner about your vision for how the two of you will share the work and how you plan to communicate. I will share an exercise later in this chapter to help the two of you frame things up so you have some clear ideas written down to keep you both honest and focused on the promises you made to each other.

When Your Partner Is the One Doubting... Eeek!

It's important to point out that you might not be the only one having doubts about your relationship right now; your partner may have their own concerns. Your partner may be wrestling with two quite emotionally charged questions: (1) Will I get lost in the mix of the "baby crazy," and (2) Am I ready to be a parent?

Too often, I see well-meaning Miracle Mamas blow the first question off a bit. It's easy to look past this very real concern and think, "Oh, he's just being a big baby. We'll figure things out." Taking that position, however, is a big mistake.

There is no denying how big of a deal finally getting pregnant after struggling with fertility is—but what I tell my mamas all the time is that your relationship came first, *and* it is the foundation of your family. Don't neglect it. Unless you want your relationship to be a statistic (and not one of the "good" ones), I can't overstate the importance of you making it clear to your partner that your relationship is the priority. If you have any desire for your family to remain intact, it must be. You and your partner are the foundation of your family (yes, I'm repeating that). The relationship you two share is the center point. Your child is an addition to the relationship. That may sound callous, but it's true.

I have seen countless situations when women lose sight of this fact, then wonder why their husbands or partners are disengaged and drift and the families they fought long and hard for begin to disintegrate. To be clear, this reality isn't just limited to male partners; it's not some foible of man. Even in same-sex couples, I see the same heartbreaking drama play out if parents don't take a good long look at their relationships and plan for the growing pains they can *reasonably* anticipate. You've got to pull your partner aside and make it clear, in no uncertain terms, that they mean everything to you and that you would appreciate their help in staying focused, as the fog and haze of motherhood in the early days is real.

Remember, you love this person enough to have a baby with them. Don't let them become relationship roadkill on the way to Mama Town. Your partner isn't weak, selfish, or ignorant just because they want love and attention. That makes them a human being! Don't forget that. When your partner knows they are the priority and knows how much you care about them, they will be less resentful of the days when your attention is solely focused on your baby. It can happen often. Therefore, getting in front of this very reasonable concern of theirs, coming up with a plan to address it, and then following through creates trust and that invaluable emotional capital that I mentioned earlier.

When it comes to the second question your partner may be wrestling with—are they ready to be a parent?—this is another place to pay close attention. Your partner may seem like the most well-adjusted, kind, loving, and even-keeled person in the world, but the enormity of the responsibility of being a parent is enough to cause anyone to second-guess themselves. I see your partner wondering about their abilities as a good thing! But, to be sure, wondering is healthy, while panic and worry can signal choppy waters ahead. Once the reality of impending parenthood sets in, this could bring up old wounds, disappointments, and maybe even memories of abuse in your partner. You are well-advised to listen carefully to what your partner has to say about their feelings and any insecurities they express. It's not easy to admit these things!

This is where listening without judgment is a wise move. Your partner's worries don't mean that they will head for the hills, so don't make their worries yours. Simply allow them to express their concerns, then acknowledge their experience and let them know how much you love them and trust that they will be a great parent—of course, only if you believe that to be true, but if you are this far in the game, my educated guess is that you do! Just be patient with them and, if it seems like they could benefit from chatting with friends or even getting the support of a coach or therapist, let them know that you will support them without judgment or pressure. Suggesting coaching or therapy from a place of anger or fear rarely works and is a breeding ground for the atom bomb in your relationship: resentment.

THE PRACTICAL

Names, Religion, and Schooling, Oh My!

Once the two of you move past the emotional questions that can come up on either side, there are always those nagging "practical" questions that you've got to face—like your baby's name, religion, or school, or the pressure of familial expectations— lurking in the background. Maybe your in-laws are dead set on your baby having a certain name and you can see an epic battle off in the distance. Perhaps everyone on your side of the family has been baptized into a specific religion that you feel no particular connection to, yet one of your parents is acting like it will besmirch your family's reputation for five generations if you deviate. Whatever the case may be, it's important that you remember your authority as Mama Bear.

Again, this is not about dominating anyone or casting aside anyone's feelings, but the bottom line is that you are the steward of this blessing—no one else. You and your partner are this child's parents. Your child deserves to be treated as an individual, not just as some cog in the wheel of generational expectations and tradition. That's not to say that traditions are bad, but there is something to be said for honoring who this child will be—separate from what others may want them to be.

Make the point of bringing these specific topics up with your partner so that the two of you can be on the same page, you can work out any kinks, and you can find effective ways to navigate through this time. As I mentioned earlier, I will be introducing an exercise shortly that you can do together to sketch out your approach to these and other topics as a couple.

The Dollars and Cents of It

Another point that I believe is important to make when it comes to this pregnancy and your relationship is the mindset that you two have when it comes to abundance. Back in chapter 5, I referred to the Abundant Pregnancy Mindset. I shared that concept because when you are the recipient of a miracle, you tend to begin to see the world in an entirely new way. You see *possibility*. You see that there is more than enough. You see opportunity in a whole new way. Having beaten the odds on this journey, you can see that *it is* possible for you to have your desires met and that your investment in this process has been more than worth it. That feeling will only grow when you hear your baby's heartbeat for the first time, and it will deepen further still the first time you feel them kick.

Your spirits are high, Mama! Your partner, on the other hand, can probably appreciate the idea of a miracle, but they may also be more focused on bills and the money spent in order to get here. There is likely part of them that wants to constrict because now you must worry about childcare, medical bills, college, and a host of other things that can send people who haven't done the work of developing an abundance mindset into a spiral. You may have wild Restoration Hardware dreams for your nursery, while your partner is thinking IKEA at best!

I want you to rest assured that this is not the end of the world. Even if your partner is relatively chill about your finances, it's important to understand that, as a society, we have generally been conditioned to clamp down and skimp in the face of uncertainty. There's nothing wrong with being wise about your investments (obviously), but who's to say that an elaborate nursery, which will one day be your baby's room as they grow, is a bad way to celebrate a miracle? You don't have to fall into societal "norms" about what you should and should not invest in and where. "Normal" is typically boring, and rarely is it an ecstatic celebration of the miraculous.

You can gently lead your partner to see things your way by sharing with them why whatever "extravagant" thing you desire makes sense. I know those words may sound a bit oxymoronic, but remember, you are Mama Bear, and you are living a reality that, at times, you doubted would come to fruition. Just tell your partner why this is important to you and what makes your heart sing about it, and share ideas with them about *how* the two of you can make it happen with ease.

Conversations are always more fruitful when you come bearing solutions rather than just complaining about your partner's inability to see things your way. When you refuse to buy into your partner's fear and instead focus on possibility, the high energy is infectious in the best possible way. Chances are that they will come around.

A SHOUT-OUT TO SINGLE MOTHERS BY CHOICE

I know that there may be some women reading this book who are Single Mothers by Choice (SMBCs), and I want to show you some love here. You might be thinking, "Gee, thanks Rosanne, finally giving me a mention here," but I want you to know that I have a special place in my heart for SMBCs. I am putting this section here simply because it makes sense, and you deserve to have a special callout. You see, I get it, sister. As an SMBC, you are doing "both" jobs. You are on your own, supported by friends and family, which is beautiful, but it is different. This means that you've got to become extremely adept at taking care of yourself.

Having coached SMBCs through conception and pregnancy, I've seen how difficult it can be, even with help from an army of friends, family, and professionals. I want to acknowledge you by encouraging you to take care of yourself, not just by having help, but by remembering that you are having your baby on your own for a reason. This is a conscious, empowered choice! While other people would run from this idea, you love yourself and your vision enough to not be trapped by convention. Nicely done! Chances are, there will be times when you wonder if you have taken on too much, but when that happens (and it will), just take a deep breath and think about the courage you had to stand by your dreams. It's a testament to your strength and willingness to listen to your heart, not to the jackals that were all too willing to tell you you're crazy.

If all this "partner" talk even gave you momentary pause, I ask you to remember this: the muscle you flexed to call in your baby is the same muscle you will use to call in the most wonderful partner, if you ever choose to do so. There is something magical and inspiring about someone who held out for their desires and brought them to fruition on *their terms*. You will attract a partner who will love and celebrate your discernment and be honored to be part of your life.

A TALE OF TWO RELATIONSHIPS: ONE GOES SIDEWAYS, THE OTHER GETS BETTER

I have shared stories of triumph to this point, so I'm going to change it up by sharing two stories to demonstrate the contrast of what can happen if you don't get on the same page with your partner and get into the habit of being honest about your wants and needs. Don't worry, it's nothing scary, but it will get a fire under your butt about having a powerful conversation.

Jana was a woman in my Fearlessly Fertile Method program. She had met and fallen in love with the man of her dreams, and there was nothing she wanted more than to have a baby with him. Having a life with him felt like a dream come true. But what she didn't realize is that he had grave reservations about two things: (1) how having a baby would impact their relationship, and (2) whether she would "let herself go" once she was pregnant.

I know that, as you read those words, you may want to stab this mystery man in the head, but hear me out. His concerns are valid. He, like everyone else, had the right to live the way he wanted to live and to get his needs met. Indeed, he may sound shallow and insecure, but there's no law against that. While Jana tried to keep up appearances, the truth is that she couldn't have been more opposite of her husband. She wasn't into the flashy lifestyle he craved. She desired a family and longed to gently glide into a more earthy, settled, and home-focused version of herself. They were on a crash course to disaster.

Truth be told, with a parade of red flags waving furiously, Jana could have easily sailed past his toxicity and on to a man who would love her without condition, *but she chose to avert her eyes.* She chose to care more about what others thought than about what *she* thought. She clung to the labels others put on her about her "advancing age" and running out of time. She felt left behind in her friend group—because she didn't have the family everyone else had. She cared more about pleasing her husband than she did about listening to the voice inside of her telling her to run.

It's no surprise that Jana struggled to conceive, and, when she did, the rainbows and unicorns she dreamed of were more like storm clouds and old nags. As much as she loved her baby, her pregnancy was misery. She agonized over being "perfect" and not gaining too much weight because she feared being "undesirable" to her man.

Once her baby was born, things did not get better. Suffice it to say that had Jana been clearer about her desires and what she truly valued, they could have had a better chance to grow closer and find more common ground. As of this writing, they are still together and trying to make things work. Jana's story serves to underscore the importance of being clear about who you are in your relationship before, during, and ultimately after your pregnancy. While Jana's dream of having a baby with her husband came true, it came at a price that she may be paying for many years to come. Bottom line? You and your baby deserve to have all the love and support in the world. Never settle for anything less.

On the other hand, there's Lina and Jonathan's story. This adorable couple met at work. Both are physicians, and their chance meeting was the stuff of a well-written rom-com for legitimately smart people with a romantic side. If you saw their pictures together, yes, you might want to barf because they are so stinking cute, but their relationship was put to the test during their fertility journey.

Both Lina and Jonathan worked grueling schedules. They did their best to sleep, eat well, and take care of themselves, but with their training in medicine, they began to worry about their dream of being parents ever coming true. When Lina came to me, she was deeply devoted to conceiving naturally, as she and Jonathan wanted to hold fast to their faith and believed a miracle could be delivered to them.

My work with Lina centered around developing a mindset open to miracles, allowing her to receive from Jonathan and to make decisions based in possibility, not fear. As Lina began shifting her mindset, she noticed that Jonathan had some catching up to do. He was more focused on "statistics," while she had moved past them. He encouraged her to take some medications, while she insisted on sticking to prayer and her carefully curated diet. While indeed this created some conflict for them, Lina summoned her Mama Bear energy and lovingly led Jonathan by sharing what was important to her and letting him truly "see" her. By being open with Jonathan, she discovered that he was scared!

Due to their openness and honesty, Lina and Jonathan's relationship was strengthened and expanded. They trusted each other more than ever before. It was clear to me that their relationship was not just resilient, but ready for their baby. Then, on Thanksgiving, less than one year after we started working together, Lina sent me her positive pregnancy test.

Lina and Jonathan continued to apply the principles that I had taught them throughout the pregnancy. They worked constructively through questions about healthcare choices and family boundaries. Hearing how this goodness served them not only in getting pregnant, but in navigating their pregnancy, had me grinning like the Cheshire Cat. And, as of this writing, their son just turned one. This family is living proof of what's possible when parents are as committed to each other as they are to having their baby.

WHO ARE WE AS WE BECOME THREE?

My goal has been to share some hard-won wisdom that will keep you focused on the fact that you, as Mama Bear, get to set the ground rules in your intimate relationship. You have a unique worldview as "the pregnant lady," which deserves to be respected in your couple. You and your partner have not been in this place together before; this is a new pregnancy and a new time. You've never needed each other more.

Give yourselves a chance to communicate openly. Take responsibility for consciously choosing who you two will be as you become three! To help you do exactly that, to close out this chapter, I will give you an exercise that I call **Who Are We as We Become Three?** The point of this exercise is to plan in advance and to do your best to avert disaster by agreeing ahead of time how you and your partner will face the wonderfully exciting challenges that await as your pregnancy progresses. Simply follow the instructions below:

- Plan a time to spend *twenty minutes uninterrupted* with your partner to complete this exercise. Limiting this conversation to twenty minutes will keep the two of you focused and the conversation moving forward. You would be wise to set a timer on your phone or oven. Just be sure to set the phone aside so you have each other's undivided attention.
- Grab a sheet of paper to write on and something to write with.
- Remember, there are no right or wrong answers to these questions. There are only *your* answers as a couple. Keep your hearts and minds open as you move through the list!

1. Now that we are pregnant, how do we choose to be more *aware of and attentive to* each other's needs?
2. Specifically, what would make Mama Bear feel super loved and supported?
3. Specifically, what would make Papa Bear feel super loved and supported?
4. When it comes to sex and intimacy, what feels right to us during this pregnancy?
5. How will we communicate without shame or judgment when it comes to sex and intimacy?
6. Regardless of any cultural or familial expectations, how do we choose, as a couple, to share information about this pregnancy with our friends and family?
7. Separate from any cultural or familial expectations, what are the boundaries we choose to have when it comes to discussions about planning for this child's

birth, this child's name, and visits with family during this pregnancy?

8. How do we choose to let each other know—without judgment or shame—that we need more support? (This speaks to the support you desire from each other, as those needs may change.)

9. How can we support each other to grow in confidence when it comes to the subject of parenting?

10. How do we choose to approach disagreements with friends or family, or when a boundary needs to be enforced?

11. What vision do we have for this miracle baby's nursery—and what excites us about it? (Also discuss how you can bring that vision to life.)

12. What is the promise that we make to each other now, as our "we" becomes three?

You are encouraged to keep the answers to these questions somewhere that you both can see them.

This time in your lives is both exciting and full of opportunities for growth. Be patient with each other and remember that you decided to have this baby because you love each other! Revisit your answers often and allow this to be a document that evolves along with you. The most important consideration in all of this is what is going to make this new family of yours happy —and what you can do to thrive. Your "we" is becoming three!

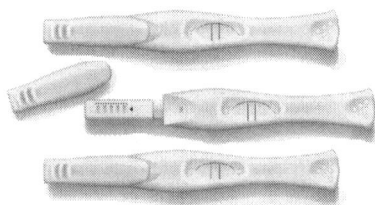

Chapter 8

Past the Goalpost, Headed toward the Finish Line

U p to this point, we've talked a lot about dealing with some of the fear, negativity, anxiety, and relationship challenges that can show up as you make your way through the early part of your Miracle Mama pregnancy. I know it can be as exciting as it is stressful, but the good news is that there will be a moment when you truly settle into the reality that you are pregnant, things are going great, and it feels like you can breathe. As unimaginable as that may seem, particularly when it feels like there's so much at stake, *it will come*—unless of course you are super committed to being miserable. But, if you're reading this book, that's probably not the case. No, you're looking forward to taking your hands off the wheel a bit and enjoying this experience!

SECOND TRIMESTER AND BEYOND: THE TRAINING WHEELS ARE OFF

At this point in your pregnancy, the name of the game is forward-focused, positive momentum. There will be more space between your prenatal appointments, and the "training wheels" of appointments every couple of weeks will be taken off. You will need to rely on your inner resources more to keep your anxiety over any uncertainty to a minimum. Smart Mamas, like you, will fill the time wisely, with soul-nourishing practices such as meditation, gentle pregnancy-appropriate exercise, time with friends, getting to know local mom groups that you may want to become part of, working on the nursery, and even beginning to look at daycare or preschools that you may want your baby to attend. You will want to get into a nice rhythm and daily routine of self-care as your energy returns, you feel more confident having crossed the twelve-week threshold for the miscarriage "danger zone," and your pregnancy symptoms have calmed down a bit.

I think of the second trimester as the "cute pregnant lady" phase. It's the time when it's more obvious that you are pregnant, you've got a cute little bump growing, you are more energetic, and you feel freer than ever to shout your joy from the rooftops. It is truly a magical time. I encourage you to absolutely bask in the glory of this moment!

The only interruptions to your bliss are likely to be some of the more important health scans for your baby, which come at the twenty-week anatomy scan and the additional scans you will have closer to thirty-two weeks to confirm that your baby's lungs and other organs are continuing to grow on schedule. I know that these appointments can be nerve-racking because we fear that the bubble of our bliss will burst if it is revealed that something is awry. If you are feeling any of those feelings, you are not alone. They're part of being a good mom and wanting the best for your baby. Where the wheels fall off is if you allow that well-founded concern to slip into full-blown anxiety and panic. Flooding your baby with stress hormones isn't awesome, so I would propose a different approach. It's the one I used while pregnant with Asher. Since we conceived him naturally, we didn't go through all the testing that is often done on embryos prior to transfer with IVF. I did have all the genetic testing once I was pregnant, and that testing said he was at a very low risk for any defects, but the fact remains that you don't know for sure until you see with your own two eyes and have the assistance of medical professionals around you.

THE POWER OF PRESENCE AND KNOWING YOUR BABY IS SAFE

There is one caveat to what I just said above, though. You don't necessarily *need* other people to tell you that your baby is safe. You can know that through the spiritual connection you feel with this child.

Truth be told, I knew in my soul that Asher was perfectly fine. I knew to the core of my being that he was healthy. I know that that may sound a little far "out there," but it's true. You don't even need to be a particularly religious person to feel this. You and this baby share a physical and spiritual connection that you've only shared with one other human being: your mom! It may sound trite, but it is true; there's no connection like the one between a mother and her child.

I'm not sharing this to proselytize any specific set of spiritual beliefs to you. I'm sharing it to acknowledge what you might already feel, so you can lean into it in the moments when you might feel a bit stressed or nervous. Truth resonates, and you can feel it in your body. When you embrace this reality, you develop trust in the internal knowing that you possess now, and you also develop trust in the power that brought this miracle baby to you—whatever you choose to call that power.

The approach I used to calm my Mama Bear nerves during the scans I went to later in my pregnancy is what I call **Presence in the Process**. The practice is simple. As I leaned back during the scans—including the anatomy scans, tests for Braxton Hicks, my glucose challenge test, and anything else that threatened to bring me anxiety over my health or Asher's—I would simply soften my gaze and ask, "What is my sweet baby showing me?" By shifting my focus away from *me* and into the present moment so that I could see what was being shown to me, I replaced my anxiety with curiosity. I made the moment about letting Asher show me if anything needed attention. (Remember: something "needing attention" is not the same as an emergency. We love to jump to unnecessary conclusions!)

Notice my choice of words in this description. It wasn't about *me*; it was about being open to what my baby wanted me to know. I would just gently talk myself through the scan, asking Asher, *"Sweetheart, what do you want to show me here? Show me your heart is healthy. Show me what your lungs look like. Show me your fingers and toes. Show me that beautiful, healthy brain of yours! Show me all the things you want me to know!"* Talking with Asher and being present brought me so much peace and connected me so deeply to him that any shred of fear I had would quickly transform into peace and awe. I strongly encourage you to practice Presence in the Process with your baby. You will be amazed at how different you feel.

We tend to exacerbate our anxiety by making circumstances about *us*, what's possibly wrong with *us*, and what will happen to *us* if something goes "wrong." Mama Bear, let me lovingly reiterate, *this pregnancy isn't about you.* It's about your baby, their health, and their well-being. As this child's mother, it's your job to be a good steward of this incredible blessing.

Sometimes people get upset when I point that out, but it's true. As emotionally mature adult women, the sooner we accept this reality, the less anxious we will be. If your baby is unwell and needs support, these scans will let you know. Your job is to be present and open to what they show you, and then to be lovingly proactive if additional attention is needed. Might this be scary? Sure. But welcome to motherhood!

You can even use Presence in the Process when it comes to doing "kick counts" and any other practices your care team suggests during your pregnancy. I take the position that Presence in the Process takes us out of living in our past "failures" and yanks us back from future-tripping—two of the primary culprits in our anxiety. The more time we spend in the present, the more we can see that we have every reason to trust in the health of our baby and in our ability to respond to anything that comes up that needs our attention. There is a softness that comes with being open to the idea that, if your baby needs help, they will let you know, in one way or another.

BUT ROSANNE, WHAT IF SOMETHING IS WRONG?

Your heart may be screeching, "Rosanne, but if there's something wrong, what do I do? What if my fear is well-founded?" Having supported clients through such scenarios, I will tell you what I told them: stay present. (As if you haven't heard me say that over and over again! But it is that important.) Sometimes we get so wrapped up in a fugue state of fear that we can't hear or process the information we are given. We immediately direct our attention to scenarios of woe and despair instead of staying present to hear exactly what the issue is and make clearheaded decisions based on that information. Yes, things can and do go wrong at later stages of pregnancy. It is devastating. But you can't possibly be who you and your baby need you to be when you let fear distract you from what's true and needed in the moment.

One of the questions that plague us when something does go wrong is, "Did I do the right thing? Did I make the right choice?" Staying present allows you to answer that question with confidence. You understood the information you were given, you connected with your baby and your intuition, and you took action like a Mama Bear. That is all anyone could be expected to do, even in the most tragic of scenarios. We tell ourselves that if something "really" bad happens, we won't recover—but you will, unless you make the choice to stay in misery.

I don't want to belabor this point because the chances of the tragic happening, absent some other information, are remote. *Stay present.* Should you find yourself in a place where additional resources are needed, let the power of presence be your flotation device until the Coast Guard arrives. There are loads of resources available for processing grief, so if that is a bridge you must cross, you will be well provided for. In the meantime, stay present.

THE POWER OF PRESENCE HELPED THESE MIRACLE MAMAS: MICHELLE AND JAMIE

The strength of this practice brings to mind the stories of two of my clients: Michelle and Jamie. My beloved Michelle had struggled with her fertility for years, enduring many rounds of IVF, multiple embryo transfers (including donor transfers), and heartbreaking miscarriages. When she got and stayed pregnant with her miracle son, we had our work cut out for us.

After having been through so much pain, Michelle understandably had high anxiety over her son's health and her ability to carry him to term. One of the skills we worked on together was staying present during all the critical points in her pregnancy—at each scan, before she could feel him kick, at all her tests, and even in preparation for his birth. I encouraged her to lean into trusting herself and this precious boy who she never gave up on.

Michelle was eventually able to find her footing in her pregnancy so she could enjoy this chapter in her life. One of the bravest women I have met in my practice, she had certainly earned her well-deserved peace! It brought me so much joy to see the transformation in her—the once exhausted and weary mama-in-the-making could now see that she was worthy of the good she desired in her life and allowed herself to receive (there's that word again!) the blessing of her son. Michelle's baby boy was born healthy, and she and her family are thriving.

My lovely lady Jamie came to me after struggling with PCOS and endometriosis. A bold spirit who refused to live her journey like a victim, Jamie had decided that she was going to make her dream of being a mom come true. Within months of completing my Fearlessly Fertile Method program, she was pregnant via IVF. As she puts it, she "crushed" IVF. She refused to let the process destroy her or her marriage. *And,* to her surprise, not only did she get pregnant, but something happened that only 2% of women ever experience: her transferred embryo split into twins. Not only was Jamie having a baby... *she was having twins!* This meant that staying present and not slipping into a panic over this very rare occurrence was critical. Jamie focused on her gratitude for this double blessing and kept herself connected to her miracle twins, practicing Presence in the Process.

(If you want to hear Michelle and Jamie share their stories in their own words, you can see their interviews on my YouTube channel. Jamie's can be found here—https://youtu.be/1sD-d3qkbfEs—and Michelle's can be found here—https://youtu.be/PuPqobnNq3U.)

PEOPLE LOVE TO SHARE HORROR STORIES—HARD PASS!

In addition to taking on the practices and ideas I have shared here, one of the wisest things you can do to protect your peace as your pregnancy progresses through your second and third trimesters is to stay away from anything or anyone peddling late pregnancy "horror stories." As well-intentioned as they may be, for some odd reason, people (and some very popular books) *love* to share harrowing stories about what could go wrong. It's as if people thrive or feed on worst-case scenarios.

Stay as far away from those stories as you can, Mama. Avoid those chapters in pregnancy books and stay the hell away from pregnancy message boards or groups that have a propensity to deal in fear porn. There's always someone in those groups who wants to share a story about a "friend of a friend" who had the unthinkable happen to them. *Nope! Delete!* Plug your ears, close your eyes, and run away. None of that is serving you! Nor is it denial to reject such slop. If you need medical advice or want to address any concerns, the words of an anonymous user who goes by the handle "BabyDust6789" (any connection to a real user going by that name is purely coincidental) are a shaky authority at best and fearmongering at worst! Words to live by: *if it leads with fear, reject it!* You will know if something is wrong, and, if so, you will get the help you need. You don't need anything that will disturb your peace and take your attention away from your healthy, happy baby.

Don't hesitate to stop people in their tracks if they even begin to share some tale of terror or woe. Simply say, "It's important for me to protect my peace during this pregnancy. I'd rather not share in that story. I'd love to talk about something else." This might seem "confrontational" to some, but remember what we've talked about: you are Mama Bear.

Let these final months and weeks of your pregnancy be about stepping into your own, Mama. This is a place where you get to really allow yourself to enjoy and embrace your pregnancy. Give yourself the gift of presence, peace, and well-deserved pampering.

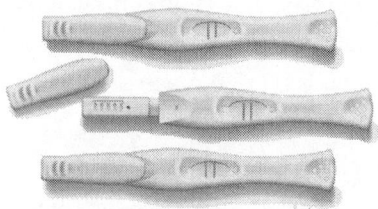

Chapter 9

Be "That" Pregnant Lady

I know we have talked about a lot of heavy topics at this point, so here's where it's about to get super fun (but no less challenging). You see, with all this new awareness you have gained, this is the point where you get to experience the magic in the execution. You have big dreams and desires for this miracle family you are building. This is the time in your life and in your pregnancy when you get to lean back and truly enjoy what you've created. No guilt. No shame. Just well-earned satisfaction.

Let me remind you that where you are today is truly the result of your obedience to the calling in your heart. It's a wondrous thing to behold. You're standing in a place few have the guts to tread. As you've discovered through our work here, you became the woman who didn't give up. Now you get to celebrate this truth with the most glorious celebration of all. You get to be "that" pregnant lady: confident, fabulous, engaged, self-aware, excellent at taking care of herself, and blissfully committed to enjoying every moment of this pregnancy.

The old you might think this sounds too good to be true, but, as you've learned—not just in this book, but certainly on the journey to your beat-the-odds baby—"too good" is simply a matter of perspective... one that, by the end of this chapter, I encourage you to drop and never pick up again, ever.

YOU GET TO BE BOUGIE

I'm a firm believer in the notion of *go big or go home,* so let me start by inviting you to do something that I know deep down you long to do: be the "bougie" pregnant lady. When I say "bougie," I mean let yourself bask in the indulgence of unapologetic consumption of all the fancy-schmancy things you fantasized about having when you were pregnant. Don't act like you don't know what I'm talking about! We see images of gorgeous pregnant women plastered all over social media with beautiful maternity clothes, buying drool-worthy decorations for their nurseries, pushing posh strollers with dangerously delectable designer diaper bags, going on glorious babymoons, and indulging in a host of other delights reserved for those celebrating the arrival of their little ones. This isn't about being materialistic. It's about giving yourself the exact kind of experience that you've longed for.

I know the temptation here is to feel like even getting to "this" place is beyond your wildest dreams, but here's where you get to push yourself all the way into the end zone for a touchdown. Be bougie, Mama!

It's true that what one considers bougie will, of course, vary, but don't overthink this. I'm willing to bet that you have some notion of what "bougie" might look like to you. For me, it was cute clothes from a chic maternity boutique that I would pass by on the regular at a decidedly bougie outdoor shopping center in the San Francisco Bay area where we lived when I was pregnant with Asher. It makes me cringe to admit this, but truth be told, I even made a point of buying a couple of the same cute dresses that the Duchess of Cambridge wore during her pregnancy with Prince George! The antiestablishment punk rock side of me is confounded by that move, but the girly girl in me saw it as a giddy masterstroke.

Whatever the bougie move is for you, make it. Treat yourself to every convenience, indulgence, and high-maintenance bougie thing you've desired, as you won't ever live this same moment again. Make it blindingly bougie. Indeed, you may go on to have another baby, but that will be an entirely different child and, therefore, a different experience. Make the most of this pregnancy by being your version of bougie *now*.

MAMA SAYS "YAAAAS!"

This may sound reminiscent of what we discussed in chapter 5 when we talked about receiving. That is intentional. The topic of allowing yourself to have what you desire is so critically important that I am approaching it from several different angles. As a mom, you will be pulled in more directions than ever before, and the pace of your life will pick up dramatically. Your ability to name, claim, and not defame your needs will be critical to your happiness and your feeling of fulfillment as a mom. The more unapologetic you are, the better.

I am also seeking to help you normalize this perspective because, in the end, you are the only one who can give yourself permission to get your needs met. It's not your partner's job, nor is it anyone else's. It's up to you, Mama. Who better to be the grantor and *guarantor* of your happiness?

To help you take receiving and bringing your desires to fruition to the next level, I have a fun exercise to share with you. It's called **Mama Says "Yaaaas!"** The process is simple:

- Grab something to write with and write on.
- Create five lines, numbered 1 through 5.
- You will be writing five sentences that begin with "I give myself permission to…"
- Finish each sentence with a precise and concise statement of the exact permission you give yourself when it comes to receiving the things/experiences that you've identified you want to receive. It's quite possible that, through the encouragement to be "bougie," you have found a few new things that you desire to receive. Give yourself the additional permission you "need." Don't feel confined to whatever you wrote in chapter 5's section on Reveling in Ridiculous Receiving; there may have been a few bougie goodies you've thought about along the way!
- You may find that you need to give yourself permission to feel and behave abundantly, even when your partner doesn't quite "get it." Give yourself specific permission to not attend family gatherings that you just don't want to attend. You might want to give yourself permission to be "needy" for the first time in your life! Whatever permission you desire, grant yourself that grace in one of those five lines.
- I encourage you to stick with five general permissions. You don't need more. As the maker of your own rules, you can probably make anything fit within the structure of those five.
- Extra credit: If you are feeling particularly frisky, give yourself permission to make "mistakes," and when

you do have the occasional "mess up," just blame it on pregnancy brain—*who could possibly fault you?*

For some, this exercise will be the permission they had been praying for, while others may run from this exercise like someone just kicked over a hornet's nest. There's no right or wrong way to do this. There are simply actions and their results. This is your chance to really claim what you desire and to give yourself the permission you need to get it.

If this exercise makes you uncomfortable, good. That's a trusty indicator that growth is needed in this area. If this exercise was "easy" for you, take it a couple steps further—where's a place in your life where you don't think you have permission? Challenge it. Maybe that's where the work is for you. Maybe it's with your partner. Wherever that place is, start testing the waters and, when you are ready, take the leap.

In the end, no one but you gives you permission to be truly happy. Regardless of what your Saboteurs may be saying right now, Mama Says "Yaaaas!" is about feeding your soul, allowing yourself to enjoy the pleasures of being in a material world without guilt or shame, and ultimately modeling to your family that Mama will not be neglected or lost in the mix. Can you see why receiving and saying "Yaaaas!" is so important? Consider it an investment in your family's happiness.

In chapter 5, I introduced the idea of Pregnant Privilege, but now is the time when I am wholeheartedly encouraging you to put it to work in your life. Mama, start taking the breaks you desire. Get someone else to carry your groceries. Ask your partner to start making more meals; your body is not only growing a baby, but you will soon be catapulted into a reality where you will give birth, start the process of healing, start feeding your baby, and survive on mind-blowingly small amounts of sleep. *You are basically beginning to perform like an elite athlete!* Start exercising your privilege. If you don't feel like walking from the farthest spot in a parking lot, tell whoever is driving that you prefer to be dropped off. Decline invitations that don't excite you—you're pregnant! Who the heck is going to blame you? Want to lay around in bed all morning? Knock yourself out! Just say no to your mother-in-law's boring invitation for tea, or the obligatory family barbecue that makes you long for air raid sirens. Stay home! Or better yet, book yourself a pregnancy massage. You know you promised yourself you'd make yourself a priority. Do it.

All of this is part of being "that" pregnant lady. You know, the one who everyone wishes they could be? Self-assured, clear about what she wants, and unapologetic about getting her needs met? Yeah, that one. She is you... if you dare to be her. (If you need to, review the five permissions you just gave yourself!)

This is also the perfect time to flex your mindset for abundance. In chapter 5, I presented you with the concept of the Abundant Pregnancy Mindset. This mindset is all about recognizing the gift that you have been given in this miracle pregnancy and using it as a basis for expanding what you believe is possible in this life. By receiving what is perhaps the most precious gift anyone can receive, in the face of what were likely quite challenging odds, you have the unique experience and authority to believe *anything* is possible. This, by its very nature, allows you to transcend the limitations that many live by when it comes to time, money, opportunity, love, experience, and the generous nature of GUS (God/Universe/Source).

Part of being "that" pregnant lady is tuning into this mindset consistently. I see the blessing of this baby as the catalyst for you to live by an entirely new paradigm. It is with this in mind that I believe you are well-equipped to silence the Saboteurs that may be coming up for you, particularly as you read this chapter. Some might blow off what I'm sharing with you here as materialistic pandering, but frankly, they are fools. They live according to a reality that, by right of your miracle pregnancy, you no longer inhabit. As the recipient of miracles, you see miracles where others see lack and limitation. Your willingness to believe in the seemingly "impossible" got you to this place; don't stop now. Stay in a place of possibility and look for opportunities everywhere to keep growing this belief in abundance. We are spiritual beings having a physical experience in a material world—you get to enjoy material things, abundantly! There is more than enough for you, Mama. Enjoy this.

EMBRACE THE CHANGES IN YOUR BODY

Expanding your consciousness so you can be "that" pregnant lady also includes keeping your body image strong as your body changes during this pregnancy. Much like you are growing past your old beliefs about what's possible in this life, you are also going to quickly realize that one of the side effects of pregnancy can be sometimes-dramatic changes to your body. I'm not just talking about weight gain, but also becoming more easily fatigued, fitting your clothes differently, and maybe even not being able to exercise or do the physical things you love to the same degree.

As much as you revel in the fact that you are pregnant, sometimes there can be fear around the bodies we've known for decades changing in big ways. With celebrities splashed all over social media flaunting their post-baby bodies bouncing back within what is alleged to be "days" after birth, it's easy to develop some unhealthy ideas around our bodies and pregnancy. These unrealistic and unquestionably "altered" photos only perpetuate unreasonable expectations for women when it comes to their bodies during and after pregnancy. This in and of itself can threaten to steal moments of joy on this journey. Reject the temptation to fall into that trap.

How this shows up on your journey can be sneaky, so be mindful. It may be a negative thought you have pop up when you see your bump truly "bumping" for the first time in the mirror. Or maybe what you will feel is dark pangs the first time you try to put on your old jeans and they don't fit. You might even experience it when you notice softening in the features of your face and even new curves around your legs, hips, and booty. This pressure of perfectionism can rob women of the wonder of seeing their bodies change. The truth is, whether anyone has mentioned it or not, your body won't ever be quite the same post-baby. That's neither good nor bad. It's just different! Your hips may change, your shoe size may change, and you may carry your post-baby softness for longer than you expect. Allow this to be okay!

I must admit that going up half a size in my shoes was a permanent change in my body that I hadn't quite anticipated. I mourned the new uselessness of my beloved Manolo Blahnik collection—but that's where my Abundant Pregnancy Mindset kicked in and reminded me that this was an opportunity for a whole *new* collection. See how awesome this mindset stuff is and how quickly it can turn proverbial lemons into lemonade? Be mindful of any pre-baby body image issues that you might have, acknowledge their presence, and be watchful of their attempts to distract you from your miracle. Just think, the miracle that brought you this baby will bless you with a new, stronger, and perhaps even more feminine body than ever before.

I found that my post-baby body was an invitation to redefine who I was physically and to reshape my view of beauty altogether. That's not a bad thing! It's simply a shift in values. Today, I'm no longer what I would call "skinny-fat." I'm no longer the size zero I was before I had Asher, and I am so happy about that. The woman I am today has a gym-toned body that is stronger and more flexible than ever, supported by the confidence that comes from knowing my body birthed a healthy baby. Now *that* is confidence! When you drop the outdated propaganda about what a woman's body "should" be pre- and post-pregnancy, you will find a level of freedom in and reverence for yourself that you may not have had before. Get excited!

BUH-BYE TO THE WANNABE

As you settle into being "that" pregnant lady, it's important to note that there can be some inner conflict about your transition from being a "wannabe" to "mama-to-be." For some, this transition will be immediate, and there may be dancing in the streets over being able to step off the fertility journey crazy train. You've graduated! But, particularly when you've had loss in the past or have hardcore fertility journey fatigue, there may be times when you feel like you're just "waiting for the other shoe to drop," as they say, so the whole idea of truly being a "mama-to-be" still feels foreign and tentative. If you find yourself in this position, review the material on receiving in chapter 5—*can you see why that was such an important chapter?* Being "that" pregnant lady is anchored in the idea that receiving is awesome... and you get to enjoy it.

The transition from "wannabe" to "mama-to-be" is up to you and how much permission you give yourself to appreciate and feel grateful in this moment. This brings me to raise a point with you that I believe is important to focus on as we discuss this transition: one of the most powerful ways you can show your gratitude for this blessing is to *enjoy it*. Not enjoying this pregnancy and forcing yourself to hold back from living it fully is what I see as fertility blasphemy. I liken it to putting plastic on your furniture! You can look, but don't touch, and certainly don't do something reckless like touch the gorgeous fabric! It basically affirms an expectation of negative experiences to come —don't do that. Not allowing yourself to fully immerse yourself in this mama experience is a form of deprivation that will only grow, because your Saboteurs will move the goalpost.

You may also find that being slow to make the transition from wannabe to mama-to-be comes from your fears around being worthy and capable. Perish the thought! You must remember that anyone who has been through what you've been through has more than proven their mettle. You have what it takes.

If you need a refresher on that subject, go back and review our work from the other chapters. Read about who you became to get here. Use this to bolster your confidence and thereby your actions. You've earned this! When you act with confidence, it builds your confidence. All this being said, give yourself permission to make the transition—you are a mama-to-be!

TAPPING INTO THE POWER OF YOUR FEMININE

Being your version of "that" pregnant lady includes keeping a close eye on your connection with the feminine energy within you. With so much happening and big changes in your body, your family, and the way you live coming, the intuitive, spiritual, creative, and self-care-oriented feminine in you may be perking up more than usual. As a hard charger, you may feel tempted to go back to your old ways and just power through any given situation, but I want to encourage you to interrupt that pattern. "That" pregnant woman honors her needs and slows down when she needs to.

It will also be interesting to notice how your tolerances change when it comes to the people you choose to have around you and the energy you are willing to entertain. I found that, when I was pregnant with Asher, my senses about people and their intentions seemed to be heightened. I was also more intuitive and creative than I had been before that point. It was as if I had tapped into an entirely new gear that I hadn't known existed. I became more judicious about who I spent time with and what kind of media I would consume. I began nurturing myself in a way that was new, more spiritually mature, and more at ease. I encourage you to explore this as well.

With your body engaged in the nurturing of a life, one would be hard-pressed to find a clearer apex in the development of your feminine power. Let yourself write, take naps, paint, sculpt, cook, design, dance, pray, make new friends, and whatever else feels truly feminine to you. Celebrate this state! You never know what treasures may come through you. Staying connected to your feminine isn't an Earth Mama thing. It comes in many forms, so just let yours evolve. Trust that your feminine energy will be knocking, so let her flow and follow her lead.

YOU CAN LOVE YOUR MOM WITHOUT HAVING TO "BE" HER

Speaking of the feminine, I want to lean in a little closer with you when it comes to the idea of becoming a mom. I am sure that right about now your mind is racing with ideas, and there are loads of well-meaning people giving their advice and opinions or tossing books and podcast episodes in your direction. That is to be expected and probably won't let up... *ever*. Instead of going down that road, though, I want to encourage you to think about the kind of mom *you* choose to be, untethered to what other people might think or expect. Said another way, you get to create your own unique brand of motherhood, regardless of what may have been modeled to you by your own mother.

If your relationship with your mom is complicated, but at some level loving, you are certainly not alone. This is a trait I see quite often among my alpha-female Miracle Mamas. The complexity of this mother-daughter relationship can create a lack of clarity in us about our identity as mothers-to-be. That could be an entire book on its own, so suffice it to say that, when it comes to cultivating your character as a mother, as much as you love your own mom, you are not confined to the paradigm of motherhood she lived by. While this point may seem obvious from an intellectual standpoint, resolving who we choose to be as a mom isn't a brain-based choice. It's deeply emotional and sometimes steeped in our own trauma.

As a conscious woman who had to make a concerted effort to get to "this place," you have the unique vantage point of being particularly cognizant of your responsibility. I don't say that to put pressure on you. Rather, this is an opportunity for you to honor your journey by doing better than just falling into the patterns by which you were raised.

No one's experience with their mother is "perfect," even if you consider yourself to be someone who had a happy childhood. We are all human, and, ideally, the goal is to continue to improve with each generation. I strongly encourage you to make some time to really think about the traits, gifts, and traditions you actively choose to bring forward from your own mother and the less desirable behaviors or attitudes that you choose to leave behind. When considering all of this, keep in mind that this is not an indictment of your mom. Not at all. You can love your mom deeply and consciously choose to head in a different direction as a mother yourself. The standards and ideals that your mom lived by are from decades past, and they may not exactly fit your lifestyle or values. I see highly educated and professionally accomplished women beat themselves up relentlessly for not baking cookies and having lavish meals prepped for their families—completely forgetting that they just completed fifty-plus-hour workweeks as professionals with demanding careers! Comparing your experience to that of your mother may be like comparing apples to oranges. They are both sweet, but very different.

Whatever the case may be, becoming that joyful, calm, self-assured, and blissful pregnant lady you've longed to be includes allowing yourself to let go of the expectations, rules, cultural confines, and "should"s that could rob you of the full, unique expression of motherhood that you desire. Take what you want from your experience with your mom, and leave the rest with love.

BUCKING THE STIGMA OF BEING AN "OLDER MOM"

So much of being "that" pregnant lady is about being comfortable in your own skin. One place where I see some women struggle, even if everything else is amazeballs, is with the perceived stigma of being an "older mom." This is where a great deal of the pressure we feel to have a baby by forty comes from. It's the notion that, somehow, life after forty just comes to a screeching halt and that Father Time is going to commit a strong-armed robbery on your energy, leaving you limp and lifeless for your kids. Nonsense! Rebuke that devil, Mama! It's misogynistic propaganda.

Having coached women from ages twenty-eight to fifty-two to miracle pregnancies, I can assure you that age has very little to do with your energy level. It has everything to do with your attitude and self-esteem. I've seen new moms in their mid to late forties with more energy than some thirty-year-olds who don't exercise or take care of themselves half as well! I see having a baby in your forties and beyond as the ultimate fountain of youth. Think about it: you've never had more confidence, experience, clarity, time, or money, on average, than you do now. You have an established group of friends and colleagues, and you may even finally live in a place that you find worthy of housing your miracle baby. Instead of having the stress of trying to figure things out alongside your kids, you kind of have this "adulting" thing down! Your kids are likely to see a more "together" version of you than you might have shown ten years ago.

When I think of my own experience, Asher has been a catalyst for me to be in better shape and take my health more seriously than ever before. He has inspired me to make my fifties and beyond even more fabulous than I thought they could be. I am more creative, energetic, and self-assured now than I would have dreamed of being when we first started trying to conceive him. When I look back on the woman I was back then, I thank GUS for making me wait, and, frankly, earn the chance to have Asher. While moms in their twenties might have a faster bounce back from pregnancy than you do, what you bring to the table, Mama, is a personal and emotional maturity that comes from really having to fight and scrap for your dream. You will mother with a steady hand, even in the face of mistakes, because you understand what it took to get "here." Trust me, you will have whatever energy you desire and need—because you know you are in the presence of a miracle.

Yup, you are "that" pregnant lady... and you will be "that" mysteriously gorgeous mom who is lit from within. Kick the notion of being a dried-up old prune to the curb. It doesn't apply to you, boo.

THE EMBODIMENT OF "THAT" PREGNANT LADY: DR. MARIEVE'S STORY

I want to share a quick story with you about one of my beloved Miracle Mamas who absolutely embodies the essence of "that" pregnant lady: Dr. Marieve. A sports medicine physician in Montreal, Canada, she came to me after struggling to conceive with her partner. They had discovered he had an issue with his sperm and that conception naturally would be difficult, if not impossible. As they moved through their treatments, they were met with failure after failure.

Being an adept problem solver, Dr. Marieve was willing to break out the big guns and call upon a surrogate to help them have their baby. In truth, however, Dr. Marieve longed to carry her own baby. They moved on to IVF treatments, but those failed, too.

One of the areas where Dr. Marieve and I focused was on helping her allow herself to enjoy her life and her journey. Instead of depriving her of things she loved, like sports, the occasional beer, and taking to the ski slopes on a bright and sunny day, I challenged her to indulge! This wasn't about being reckless or disregarding the advice of her physician (she *is* a physician, for Heaven's sake!); it was about letting her really *live* during this time in her life. So, in the two weeks following the embryo transfer, Dr. Marieve took to heart everything I had coached her to do. Just two days post-transfer, she went skiing and did the unthinkable: she had a beer with friends right after. I told her to show her baby who she truly was and to let her light shine so brightly that her baby could find his way home.

At the end of her glorious two-week wait, Dr. Marieve was pregnant. She had taken excellent care of herself, gotten facials, had her hair done. She had let herself live in bliss. She became "that" pregnant lady as she carried these practices through her pregnancy. She gave herself full permission to be herself, have her needs met, and be exactly who she dreamed of being while pregnant.

If you want to see her version of "that" pregnant lady, check out my interview with her on YouTube, found here: https://youtu.be/sObVeLWwack. You will see exactly what I mean.

MAMA BEAR IS THE SHOT-CALLER IN THE DELIVERY ROOM

As we close out our discussion about being "that" pregnant lady, I want to make sure that you understand that this also makes you the shot caller in the delivery room when you have your baby. "That" pregnant lady protects her peace. She holds her happiness, privacy, and sacred space with her new family in the highest regard. She refuses to tolerate guilt, shame, undue family pressure, or misplaced responsibility for others' unfounded expectations.

None of this means that you don't want to share your joy with your family, but it does consider that giving birth is one of the most intimate and vulnerable moments in your life. You will be exposed in ways you might not want to share with others. Yes, your mother-in-law might be eager to see her new grand-baby, but does she really need to see your vagina, too? Nah, babe. That might be a bridge too far.

If this is a sensitive subject, just let your partner know how you feel and ask them to honor the family the two of you have created. If that becomes a bit of a battleground, you can always enlist the support of your labor and delivery nurses or midwife. They are quite adept and very willing to tell busybody relatives to simmer down and hang out in the waiting room when relatives have stayed too long or just don't get the hint.

With that in mind, be sure you throw some lovely gifts for your delivery team in your hospital "go bag." It will go a long way toward helping you have the birth experience you truly desire.

"THAT" PREGNANT LADY IS YOU

It is my sincere prayer that what we have talked about here, when it comes to being "that" pregnant lady, has inspired you to give yourself as much license and agency as you desire to have during your pregnancy. You get to embody everything you daydreamed about before your pregnancy. Celebrate your achievement by living this time with your whole heart. Say huge yeses. Make your present during this pregnancy one of wonderment and commitment to truly being alive.

I absolutely loved who I became while I was pregnant with

Asher. Pregnancy was an experience that left an indelible impression upon me and helped me cultivate a level of self-respect that can only come from consciously choosing to live exactly as I wanted, in the midst of the dream that I brought to fruition. I learned that I could trust myself, my body, and the desire in my heart to be a mom. I also saw my relationship with my husband and other people I care about grow. My pregnancy was an incredible time of connection to my feminine side, which did wonders for my creativity and intuition. For the first time in my life, I felt truly comfortable in my skin. My hope for you is that you will feel all of these things and so much more.

Rather than blowing off what may feel like "review" to you in this chapter, see this instead as reinforcement of an urgent call to action. Being a few chapters ahead of you in this life and on my journey from wannabe to bona fide mama, I know how tempting it is to shrink back from your power and fall back into playing small in your life so that you don't shine "too bright" or become "too much" during your pregnancy. Reject the fears that may creep in. Focus instead on your gratitude for each moment with your miracle baby. Disregard what others might think. This is your time, Mama. You'll soon realize that instead of being some mystical, unattainable creature, "that" pregnant lady is just a woman who decided to be fearless. And "that" pregnant lady is you.

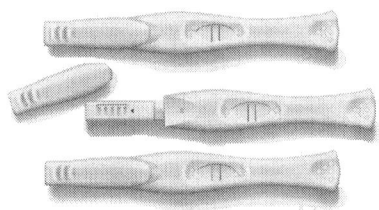

Conclusion

Live Your Fearless Pregnancy

L ove, congratulations. You have made it to what I hope is the most exciting, fun, and challenging part of the book. Yes, we've had some laughs, but now is where things get really interesting. This is where the rubber meets the road: you get to apply what I've taught you in vivo! No more theory, no more living in your head; you get to make this concept of Fearless Pregnancy your reality.

This may seem both exciting and daunting. Just remember that two things can be true at the same time, so that's not a bad thing. It's proof that you are still human! That's the thing about mindset. It doesn't make you a robot. Rather, it is an affirmation and celebration of the free will GUS gave you. Use it wisely. Decide that you will be Fearless from this moment on!

There may be a part of you that doesn't quite know exactly where to start with everything I've taught you. The answer is to begin by making the *decision* that you will be Fearless. It's just a decision. The Latin root of the word decision is literally "to cut." In our context here, that means to cut off any retreat to an existence of fear and doubt. You are Mama Bear now. You understand what it means to summon that energy, and you are well within your rights to do so!

Expect that this transition may not be easy, but make the decision that you will stay on track. If you "mess up," just make the decision that you will try again. Don't beat up the pregnant lady! Being Fearless in our lives is a constant state of practice, rather than a fixed destination. Your fearlessness will be tested on many levels, but that's nothing to be afraid of. Chances are that you may surprise yourself at how easy it is for you to recognize fear and doubt when they come up and resoundingly "pants" them like a middle school bully.

There will be those around you who might not be comfortable with this newfound confidence, ease, and joy of yours, but remember, *you* are Mama Bear, and you get to live your miracle pregnancy any way you wish. And, on that note, feel free to build and expand upon what I have shared with you here. It is a starting point. As the designer of your life, it is more important that you honor your uniqueness, rather than following any methodology with puritanical orthodoxy. That's hardly what my work is intended to be. It is for decidedly open-hearted, critical thinkers committed to growth, challenge, and living life to its most gorgeous fullness. It is my sincere wish that you will receive what I have shared here with the love with which it has been given.

While I have written this book as a guide, you may find yourself desirous of more in-depth instruction, coaching, and guidance. If that is the case, feel free to check out my website at www.frommaybetobaby.com and reach out to us. We will provide you with ideas and ways to take this work to the next level if you choose. No matter what, Mama, keep your eyes focused on the fact that this good that you have called into your life was meant for you. Show your gratitude for this blessing by enjoying everything it has to offer.

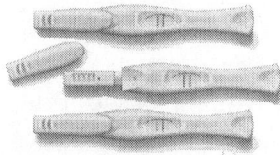

Your Fearless Pregnancy Tool Kit

To make the resources I have shared in this book easily accessible in a *break glass in case of emergency* situation, I am listing all the most vital exercises and tools here, along with the chapter in which each is found:

- Your Pregnancy Promise, Chapter 2, pages 16–18
- Woman, You Did Good Letter, Chapter 3, pages 29–30
- Pre-Scan Calming Ritual, Chapter 3, pages 31–32
- Be the Woman You Said You'd Be, Chapter 3, page 34
- Stay Present, Chapter 3, page 34
- It's You and I, Little One, Chapter 3, page 35
- Pregnancy Visioning Exercise, Chapter 4, pages 43–44
- Bust Out the Good China, Chapter 4, page 44
- Fearless Pregnancy Daily Practice, Chapter 4, pages 48–49
- Pregnant Privilege, Chapter 5, pages 58–60
- Abundant Pregnancy Mindset, Chapter 5, pages 60–61

- Reveling in Ridiculous Receiving, Chapter 5, pages 62–64
- The Velvet Rope Technique, Chapter 6, pages 67–69
- Summon Mama Bear Energy, Chapter 6, pages 78–80
- "Exorcise" the Expectations, Chapter 6, pages 79–80
- Who Are We as We Become Three?, Chapter 7, pages 101–103
- Presence in the Process, Chapter 8, pages 107–108
- Mama Says "Yaaaas!", Chapter 9, pagse 115–117

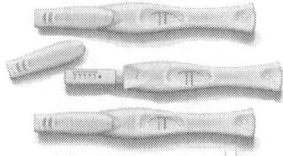

About The Author

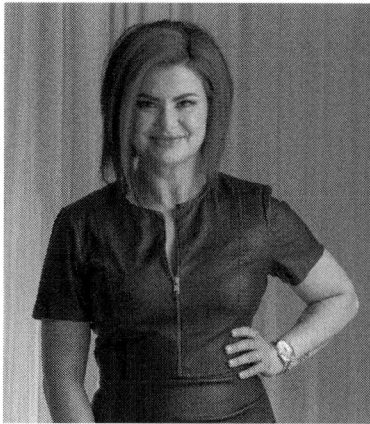

Rosanne Austin, two-time best-selling author and creator of the Fearlessly Fertile Method, is a former state prosecutor turned fertility fairy godmother. She is the fertility coach physicians trust and women around the world turn to when they are committed to mama-making success.

Rosanne overcame her own seven-year struggle with fertility and had her son naturally at almost 44, when medicine had given up on her. She is committed to helping women get and stay pregnant. With her books, podcast, online courses, and retreats, Rosanne helps her clients become the moms they were meant to be. She resides in The Woodlands, Texas, with her husband, son, two chihuahuas, and two formerly feral cats. When she's not writing, coaching, or chasing her son around, she loves traveling, deep conversation, high tea, and Jane Austen movie marathons.

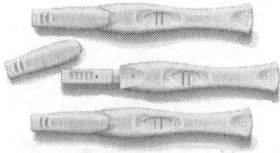

Thank You for Reading!

Want a mantra that will help you stay confident throughout your miracle pregnancy, no matter what?

I've put the empowering five-word mantra that I lived by during my miracle pregnancy on a business card-sized printable download, *just for you!*

To thank you for finishing my book, I want to share the mantra that kept me confident and grateful through every stage of my miracle pregnancy. My Miracle Mamas around the world use it too!

This printable card will keep you focused on the *five* words that will steady you in any situation that shows up on your journey.

And saying this mantra feels so good you'll want to *SHOUT IT!*

Save it to your phone or print it and tuck it into your back pocket so it's there to keep you living your pregnancy with ease and joy.

Get your FREE Fearless Pregnancy Mantra Card *now!*

Scan the QR code or go to https://www.frommaybetobaby.com/
ffp-gift-2.